Kidney Disease Management

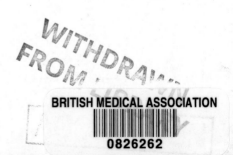

D1333595

WITHDRAWN
FROM

Kidney Disease Management

A Practical Approach for the Non-Specialist Healthcare Practitioner

Edited by

Rachel Lewis RN, RSCN, MSc, MA (Econ), BA (Hons)

Nurse Practitioner
Manchester Business School
The University of Manchester
Manchester, UK

Helen Noble RN, PhD, BSc, PG Dip Academic Practice

Lecturer in Health Services Research
Queen's University Belfast
Belfast, Northern Ireland, UK

WILEY-BLACKWELL

A John Wiley & Sons, Ltd., Publication

This edition first published 2013, © 2013 by John Wiley & Sons, Ltd

Wiley-Blackwell is an imprint of John Wiley & Sons, formed by the merger of Wiley's global Scientific, Technical and Medical business with Blackwell Publishing.

Registered Office
John Wiley & Sons, Ltd, The Atrium, Southern Gate, Chichester, West Sussex, PO19 8SQ, UK

Editorial Offices
9600 Garsington Road, Oxford, OX4 2DQ, UK
The Atrium, Southern Gate, Chichester, West Sussex, PO19 8SQ, UK
111 River Street, Hoboken, NJ 07030-5774, USA

For details of our global editorial offices, for customer services and for information about how to apply for permission to reuse the copyright material in this book please see our website at www.wiley.com/wiley-blackwell.

Library of Congress Cataloging-in-Publication Data

Kidney disease management : a practical approach for the non-specialist healthcare practitioner / [edited by] Rachel Lewis, Helen Noble.
      p. ; cm.
   Includes bibliographical references and index.
   ISBN 978-0-470-67061-3 (pbk.)
   I. Lewis, Rachel, 1965– II. Noble, Helen, 1964–
   [DNLM: 1. Kidney Diseases.   2. Chronic Disease–therapy.   3. Renal Insufficiency, Chronic.   WJ 300]
   616.6′1–dc23
                                                         2012032765
A catalogue record for this book is available from the British Library.

Wiley also publishes its books in a variety of electronic formats. Some content that appears in print may not be available in electronic books.

Cover design by: Steve Thompson

Set in 9/12.5pt Interstate by SPi Publisher Services, Pondicherry, India

Printed and bound in Malaysia by Vivar Printing Sdn Bhd

1   2013

Contents

Contributors

David Colin-Thomé

Dr David Colin-Thomé is an independent healthcare consultant and former general practitioner at Castlefields in Runcorn. He also spent several years as the National Clinical Director of Primary Care and clinical lead for the long-term conditions programme, Department of Health, England.

Emma Coyne BSc(Hons), ClinPsyD

Dr Emma Coyne is a clinical psychologist working within the adult renal unit at Nottingham University Hospitals NHS Trust. She is particularly interested in improving psychological care using compassion-based interventions. She also has a special interest in improving services and provision for young adults with CKD.

Indranil Dasgupta MBBS, MD, DM, FRCP

Indranil Dasgupta is a consultant physician and nephrologist at Birmingham Heartlands Hospital and honorary senior lecturer at the School of Clinical and Experimental Medicine, University of Birmingham. His main areas of interests are hypertension, chronic kidney disease, pre-dialysis care and renal bone disease.

Jeanette Denning RGN

Jeanette Denning is a senior sister in peritoneal dialysis and pre-dialysis pathway at the Leeds Teaching Hospitals NHS Trust.

Aileen Dunleavy MRPharmS (Ipresc)

Aileen Dunleavy is senior renal pharmacist at Crosshouse Hospital, Kilmarnock. She is co-editor of the *Renal Drug Handbook* and has been a renal pharmacist for 18 years. She is a pharmacy prescriber and has an interest in the management of anaemia.

Aisha I. Geeson MBChB, MRCP

Dr Aisha Geeson graduated from Dundee Medical School in 2006 and has worked in Edinburgh, Swansea and Bristol. She is currently a specialist registrar in renal medicine at Southmead Hospital, Bristol, having developed her interest in renal medicine while working in Morriston Hospital, Swansea.

Keith Harkins MBChB, MRCP

Dr Keith Harkins is a consultant physician and geriatrician at Wythenshawe Hospital, University Hospital of South Manchester. Within elderly care Dr Harkins is particularly interested in rehabilitation, continence and end-of-life care.

Maggie Higginbotham BSc (Hons)
Maggie Higginbotham is a renal specialist nurse currently working as clinical educator in York Renal Services. She qualified as a registered nurse in 1987, and began renal nursing in 1988 at St James's Hospital, Leeds, before moving to York Renal Services in 1999. She has recently completed a BSc in healthcare practice at the University of Leeds. Maggie is passionate about providing a high standard of multi-professional care to renal patients and their families and has a keen interest in 'user involvement'.

Rachel Hilton MA, PhD, FRCP
Dr Rachel Hilton received her BA at the University of Oxford in 1985 (physiological sciences) and her BM BCh in 1988. She has been a consultant nephrologist at Guy's and St Thomas' NHS Foundation Trust since 1999, and was lead clinician in nephrology between 2003 and 2008. She has held an honorary appointment in the School of Medicine at King's College London since 2006. She is currently R&D theme lead for transplantation and medical lead in transplantation. Dr Hilton is interested in renal transplantation, living kidney donation, viral infection after transplantation, autoimmune diseases, renal disease in pregnancy and renal disease in patients with human immunodeficiency virus.

Helena Jackson BSc (Hons), PgDip, MSc, RD
Helena Jackson is a renal dietitian at St George's Hospital, London. She has worked as a renal dietitian since 1995 in all areas of renal dietetics, from enteral and parenteral feeding to optimising patient motivation and understanding of diet. She is the co-author of two books on diet for patients with chronic kidney disease.

Sheila Johnston RN, MSc, BSc
Sheila Johnston is the lead nurse, clinical lead in chronic kidney disease (CKD) at the Royal Free London NHS Foundation Trust. She has been working within the renal specialty since 1995 and moved into specialist practice in CKD in 2003. She has a particular interest in the supportive and palliative care needs of those patients opting not to have dialysis, and in further developing shared decision making in this group to enhance their end-of-life care.

Colin H. Jones MBChB, MD, FRCP, MEd (ClinEd)
Dr Colin Jones is a consultant physician and nephrologist at York Teaching Hospital NHS Foundation Trust. He qualified in 1988 (University of Birmingham), was awarded a Doctor of Medicine degree in 1999 (University of Birmingham) and a Master's in Education in 2008 (University of Leeds). He strongly believes in providing holistic patient-centred care delivered through evidence-based medicine and supported by robust audit and governance mechanisms. He is actively involved in clinical research and in undergraduate and postgraduate education.

Lesley Lappin, RN, BSc (Hons), MSc
Lesley Lappin is a clinical nurse specialist and community dialysis lead at Salford Royal NHS Foundation Trust. She has worked in kidney care for

23 years and is the nursing lead for the peritoneal dialysis service at Salford Royal Hospital. In 2010 she was awarded a Kidney Research/BRS joint fellowship and is studying for a doctorate in quality improvement sustainability.

David Lewis MBChB, MD, FRCP

Dr David Lewis is a nephrologist and general physician. He is the clinical lead for peritoneal dialysis at Salford Royal NHS Foundation Trust and has a particular interest in multidisciplinary working.

Rachel Lewis RN, RSCN, MSc, MA (Econ), BA (Hons)

Rachel Lewis is a nurse practitioner at Manchester Business School engaged in health services research in general practice. She previously worked as a community matron and is interested in care integration and service delivery for people with multiple chronic conditions. She has spent many years working in adult and children's renal services, and worked for several years as a nurse adviser to the Department of Health, working with the renal and pathology policy teams.

Rosemary Macri

Rosemary Macri is the Chief Executive of the British Kidney Patient Association (BKPA). Rosemary first worked with the BKPA in 1977 and became a personal assistant to the founder president. Following a break to pursue other opportunities she returned to the charity in 2002, and in 2008 became its Chief Executive. The BKPA provides advice, support and financial help for people with kidney disease.

Beverley Matthews RN

Beverley Matthews is the director of NHS Kidney Care and Liver Care. Originally a nurse, she has worked for many years in renal services as a transplant coordinator and a network manager. NHS Kidney Care aims to improve the outcomes for people with kidney disease, and achieves this by helping to embed evidence-based innovations in everyday practice.

Helen Noble RN, PhD, BSc, PG Dip Academic Practice

Dr Helen Noble is a lecturer in Health Services Research at Queen's University Belfast. Previously she worked as a ward manager, matron and then as a senior clinical nurse specialist involved in setting up one of the first renal palliative and supportive care programmes in the UK. She has research expertise in nephrology nursing, particularly related to those who opt not to embark on dialysis, and their carers, and is interested in developing interventions to support this group.

Sally Noble APD, BA

Sally Noble has worked as a specialist renal dietitian in both Australia and the United Kingdom. She is currently working as a senior renal/diabetes dietitian in Brisbane, Australia. She is interested in promoting healthy balanced diets for people with kidney disease to prevent and manage their condition, as well as investigating ways to screen and manage patients with poor nutrition.

Rajib Pal MBChB, MRCGP, MRCP, DCH, DRCOG, PG Cert (Med Ed)
Dr Rajib Pal is a general practitioner in Birmingham. He is a GP trainer, foundation year 2 supervisor, undergraduate tutor and vascular and research lead clinical lead for stroke. He is also a member of the NICE Guideline Development Group for Acute Kidney Injury, and of the Department of Health Acute Kidney Injury Delivery Group.

Hugh Rayner MA, MBBS, MD, FRCP, DipMedEd
Dr Hugh Rayner is a consultant nephrologist at the Heart of England NHS Foundation Trust and clinical lead for the West Midlands Renal Network. He is interested in improving the care of people with all stages of chronic kidney disease and has a long-standing research interest in clinical nephrology, especially through the Dialysis Outcomes and Practice Patterns Study (www. dopps.org).

Charles R. V. Tomson MA, BM, BCh, FRCP, DM
Dr Charlie Tomson is a consultant nephrologist at Southmead Hospital, Bristol. He is primarily a clinician and has worked on clinical practice guidelines for the Renal Association, Royal College of Physicians, KDIGO and ERBP. He is interested in quality improvement in kidney care – how to spread the adoption of best practice, and how to support shared decision making in the care of patients with kidney disease.

Graham Woodrow MBChB, MD, FRCP
Dr Graham Woodrow is a consultant nephrologist at St James's University Hospital, Leeds Teaching Hospitals NHS Trust. He has particular interests in peritoneal dialysis, nutrition and body composition analysis in renal disease, and in the management of diabetic renal disease.

Foreword

This is a succinct, comprehensive and well-written book covering optimal care for people with kidney disease across the healthcare system. There is much here for the specialist and generalist, with the focus on the individual patient. What is generally lacking in the NHS is a systematic focus on and accounting to the patient. Similarly, there is a great deal of rhetoric about integration, but unless it produces a transparently better service for individual patients it will simply be yet another word in the bureaucratic lexicon. This publication adeptly addresses that system-wide deficit.

Care for people with kidney disease has, until recently, received insufficient attention compared with other acute and chronic conditions. There are, as ever, excellent exemplars of optimal care – but rarely across the whole system of care. For instance, the increasing challenge of managing metabolic syndrome has only relatively recently been recognised as a system-wide issue, particularly in primary care. To date, the development of locally based, community-focused integrated services, with improved access for people with the spectrum of acute and chronic kidney problems, has not been high enough in the list of local priorities.

This book is much needed and timely, given the opportunities offered by the prioritising of long-term conditions, by a future of clinicians influencing and/ or leading commissioning, and by a growing focus on clinical and patient-reported outcomes.

Congratulations to the editors and contributors. This is a good educative read for clinicians and non-clinicians alike, addressing the issues that often prevent the system-wide improvement of care. It also incidentally serves as an excellent template for publications on other long-term conditions.

Dr David Colin-Thomé
Independent Healthcare Consultant, UK

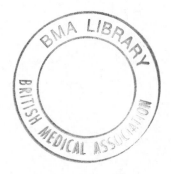

Foreword

How much easier it would be for health professionals if patients presented with just one disease! Sadly, we all know this is rarely the case, and with long-term conditions such as chronic kidney disease there are often many associated comorbidities influencing outcomes – particularly with growing numbers of elderly patients.

It's refreshing to see a book like this providing an invaluable source of knowledge and understanding about the management of kidney disease for non-specialist professionals including nurses, junior doctors, general practitioners, pharmacists and dietitians. No one can be an expert in every field, but it's important to know where to find expert opinion and advice.

This informative book has been put together with the support and input of many clinical renal experts, who have been willing to share their knowledge and years of experience, and I'm sure it will be an excellent resource for those caring for kidney patients for the first time – as well as for those with some years of experience.

Each chapter is informed by patient and family perspectives and adds a valuable practical insight into what it's like to live with kidney disease and how it impacts on daily life and families. These may be particularly useful for service design and care planning.

The British Kidney Patient Association supports local and national initiatives that improve the care and quality of life for kidney patients around the UK. I feel sure that this new information resource will help achieve these aims by enabling optimal management of patients with chronic kidney disease, encouraging improved development of personal care plans and enabling more patient choice.

Rosemary Macri
British Kidney Patient Association, UK

Introduction

Managing Patients with Chronic Kidney Disease in Non-Specialist Areas: a Chronic Illness Approach

Rachel Lewis

Manchester Business School, The University of Manchester, UK

Reasons for writing the book

The purpose of this book is to help optimise the management of patients with chronic kidney disease (CKD) across the healthcare spectrum. It is aimed at a number of non-specialist professionals including nurses, junior doctors, general practitioners, pharmacists and dietitians. It includes a number of health states and settings in which people with kidney disease are managed. In contrast to many other publications on chronic disease management, this book emphasises the multiplicity of influences on ill health and illustrates the necessity to focus on the needs of the individual, particularly within systems of care.

Many patients with established or deteriorating kidney disease will be managed by a specialist team, and this book is not intended to negate the need for specialist renal services. Instead, it highlights some practical considerations necessary to care for people with kidney problems in situations where a specialist practitioner is not always required or may not be immediately available. It provides some general principles for safe and effective care in a number of situations and settings and provides guidance on circumstances in which a specialist should be contacted. It is written by clinical staff and reflects their experiences of managing CKD. It also reflects a number of patient and family narratives, a perspective often obscured by the immediacy of acute settings. In the same way that patients are individuals, so too are healthcare staff; consequently the book includes a number of professional perspectives and styles intended to appeal to a team approach to care management. The book is written in an accessible format, aimed at busy professionals, and cites key material for further information.

1. Managing Chronic Conditions: The Policy Context

Beverley Matthews

The ageing population and the rising incidence and prevalence of chronic conditions suggest that the current organisation of health services within the National Health Service (NHS) is unsustainable. A major driver of costs within the present system is the population dependence on acute care. In response, recent healthcare policy has been directed at reducing the number of hospital beds and moving care for people with chronic conditions into the community. Historically, people with kidney disease have been cared for in different settings, partly because oflimited capacity on renal wards, but often because they have required other services such as rehabilitation, general surgery or other specialist provision. In addition, there is a growing cohort of patients with multiple chronic conditions, including CKD, who, with appropriate management, can be safely managed in primary care. Chapter 1 provides an overview of the changing context of healthcare in England: the shift from acute care to the community; the need for more general, as opposed to disease-specific, chronic care; and the current development of policy that aims to promote more integrated and collaborative ways of working.

2. What Non-Specialists Need to Know about Chronic Kidney Disease

Graham Woodrow, Jeanette Denning and David Lewis

The health needs of patients with CKD are not homogeneous and vary over time, but all CKD patients share some health issues that need to be regularly appraised if patient outcomes are to be optimised. Chapter 2 provides an introduction to the different types of renal replacement therapy (RRT), including transplantation, and illustrates some of the technical and practical issues surrounding dialysis. As well as an overview of the clinical characteristics associated with CKD (anaemia, blood pressure management and bone mineral disease), the chapter considers issues associated with particular treatment modalities.

3. A Practical Approach to Chronic Kidney Disease in Primary Care

Hugh Rayner, Rajib Pal and Indranil Dasgupta

People with CKD cover a spectrum of health states, and treatment is generally titrated around the stages of the disease, treatment decisions and individual wishes and circumstances. Chapter 3 focuses on patients with stage 1-3 CKD, who are primarily managed in general practice. The aim of care is to arrest or slow down any deterioration in renal function. This requires treatment of pre-disposing conditions such as high blood pressure and diabetes, appropriate management of inter-current illnesses, optimising vascular health and pro-moting general wellbeing through lifestyle advice and support. The chapter also considers some 'common' scenarios in deteriorating renal function and how monitoring estimated glomerular filtration rate (eGFR) over time can inform a systematic approach to identifying those most at risk. Unusually, but pertinently, the chapter includes patients with a transplant kidney in the group with CKD. As the population of patients with a transplanted kidney increases with improved survival, they will increasingly present across the healthcare system. Non-renal practitioners need to be aware of drug interactions, as well as conditions that affect the absorption of immunosuppressive medication.

4. General Considerations Related to Treatment Modalities

Aisha I. Geeson, Charles R. V. Tomson and Lesley Lappin

CKD includes a spectrum of health states, not all of which are suitable for or responsive to all forms of treatment. In addition, increasingly many older patients have a number of other chronic conditions, they may be frail and cognitively impaired, and they may live alone. Although not necessarily a barrier to dialysis, all these factors need to be considered in relation to the-likely benefits and/or burdens of treatment regimes. Chapter 4 discusses the importance of early referral to specialist services, the factors influ-encing dialysis choice, empowering patients and shared decision making. It also discusses some of the clinical contraindications to individual treatment modalities.

5. Psychosocial Aspects of Living with Chronic Kidney Disease

Emma Coyne

This book considers the management of CKD across a spectrum of health states, but for the most part focuses on people who have stage 3–5 CKD. These are people who are likely to require treatment and support for the rest of their lives. This chapter reflects the experiences of patients, partners, families and professionals. It provides an insight into the reality of living with CKD and the impact this has on quality of life, not just for patients but for their immediate families as well. Patients and their partners are often experts in their care and should be involved in planning that care, particularly in non-specialist areas. The intention is to encourage providers to consider the wider manifestations of kidney disease and how their service design can best fit the needs of patients in the context of other services such as primary care.

6. Acute Kidney Injury in Hospitalised Patients

Keith Harkins, Rachel Lewis and Rachel Hilton

Older people are more likely to have additional complications and poorer outcomes than younger adults. It is not possible, or always appropriate, to manage all patients with acute kidney injury (AKI) in specialist units. Chapter 6 focuses on the causes, diagnosis and management of AKI in people whose condition may be complicated by multiple morbidity, frailty and cognitive impairment. It assumes a non-specialist setting and provides a guide to determining the parameters of care that consider the patient's quality of life before AKI and the likely prognosis associated with various treatment options. It emphasises the importance of an ongoing dialogue with the patient (where possible) and close family members and/or carers. It stresses the need for a realistic, holistic assessment of the patient's prognosis by a senior physician and the benefits of pre-empting possible complications.

7. Management of Patients with or at Risk of Kidney Disease on the Surgical Ward

Colin H. Jones and Maggie Higginbotham

Patients admitted to hospital for reasons other than kidney disease are at an increased risk of developing an acute kidney injury. This includes people undergoing a surgical procedure. Some patient groups are at a higher risk than others, and these include patients with pre-existing chronic conditions, including CKD. Identifying those patients at risk, assessing the risks and managing them proactively reduces the likelihood of avoidable harm. Chapter 7 discusses best practice in identifying patients with, or at risk of, AKI, pre-, peri- and postoperatively. It covers the spectrum of management, from those patients with no pre-existing kidney problems to those who require maintenance dialysis. It stresses the importance of determining the extent of the patient's renal impairment and their maintenance regime. Ongoing communication with the renal specialist team is fundamental to optimising outcomes in this population.

8. Medication Management and Chronic Kidney Disease

Aileen Dunleavy

As with other aspects of managing kidney disease, medication regimes, whilst adjusted to complement general health states and treatment modalities, are tailored to the patient's individual circumstances and usually managed by a nephrologist. Chapter 8 explains some of the general principles associated with medication management and the reasoning behind them. Safe and effective prescribing for people with CKD requires information regarding the extent of renal impairment and some understanding of how the drugs in question are absorbed and excreted. This chapter includes some important resources for prescribing support in the UK.

9. Optimising Nutrition in People with Chronic Kidney Disease

Helena Jackson and Sally Noble

Diet plays an important part in preventing CKD and delaying its progression; it is also one of life's pleasures and is often restricted in patients with stage 3–5 CKD. In most instances, patients with CKD are advised to follow the same healthy-eating guide as the general population. Those with advanced disease usually require modifications to their diet, and individual dialysis modalities are associated with different restrictions, as is the case for patients who have diabetes as well as CKD. Dietary advice and support are provided by renal dietitians on an individual basis as necessary; however, patients and/or their families are generally very knowledgeable about their dietary constraints and can be a useful resource for healthcare professionals.

10. Supportive and Palliative Care for Patients with Advanced Kidney Disease

Sheila Johnston, Helen Noble and Rachel Lewis

All patients with CKD require a palliative care approach in the sense that they will never be cured. However, this chapter is concerned with those patients whose overall health is deteriorating irrespective of their treatment regime. Patients with stage 4 or 5 kidney disease have a much shorter life expectancy than those of a similar age in the general population, and for patients on dialysis it is even shorter. Chapter 10 discusses some of the practical difficulties in identifying and managing deteriorating and terminally ill patients. It illustrates the unpredictability of chronic disease trajectories and the importance (and difficulty) of being prognostically realistic.

Conclusion

This edited collection is aimed at improving the care of people with CKD. It represents 'real life' health care in which effective continuity and coordination of care are often challenged by complex and fragmented systems. Unusually, it includes professional insights into the practicalities of managing complex patients. It emphasises the centrality of the patient and family and the need to share information and expertise across traditional boundaries.

Chapter 1
Managing Chronic Conditions: The Policy Context

Beverley Matthews

NHS Kidney Care and Liver Care, UK

Introduction

The rising incidence and prevalence of chronic conditions presents a serious challenge to the effectiveness and sustainability of current and future healthcare services. A major issue is the increasing number of people with multiple chronic conditions and health services that continue to be organised around specific diseases. It is evident that chronic kidney disease (CKD) encompasses a spectrum of health states, and that these can be negatively affected by other chronic conditions and age-related problems such as memory impairment and mobility issues. Similarly, socioeconomic factors such as deprivation also adversely influence health outcomes. In effectively meeting the diverse needs of people with chronic conditions, a population management approach is required whereby the focus of care is based on the level of need and extends beyond traditional disease-specific approaches. Successive health policies reflect this shift with initiatives such as 'Our health, our care, our say' (Department of Health 2006) and the long-term conditions National Service Framework (Department of Health 2005) aimed at services being delivered through a 'whole systems approach'. Continuity of care is required across traditional organisational boundaries through more effective collaboration of professionals. Key to this approach is engaging and supporting the patient in self-management. This chapter provides an overview of the changing context of healthcare services, including the innovative work of NHS Kidney Care in working across healthcare sectors and the current policy work which supports a more integrated and collaborative approach in supporting people with chronic kidney disease.

Kidney Disease Management: A Practical Approach for the Non-Specialist Healthcare Practitioner, First Edition. Edited by Rachel Lewis and Helen Noble.
© 2013 John Wiley & Sons, Ltd. Published 2013 by John Wiley & Sons, Ltd.

Chronic kidney disease in context

The effective management of chronic or long-term conditions poses a significant challenge for healthcare systems across the world. In England, around 15 million people have a long-term condition. While the number of people in England is likely to remain relatively steady, the number of people with multiple chronic conditions is expected to rise by a third over the next 10 years. People with long-term conditions account for 29% of the population in England, but are the most frequent users of healthcare services, accounting for 50% of all general practice appointments and 70% of all inpatient bed days. It is estimated that the treatment and care of those with long-term conditions accounts for 70% of the primary and acute care budget in England. This means around one-third of the population accounts for over two-thirds of the spend (Department of Health 2011). More significant than the impact on resources is the effect that long-term conditions have on quality of life. Each year around 170 000 people die prematurely in England, with the main causes being cancers and circulatory diseases. The proportion of people with a limiting long-term condition in work is a third lower than among those without (Department of Health 2011).

Healthcare services continue to be organised around specific conditions. Even for people with a single chronic condition, care is typically provided across a number of different health professionals and organisations. The resultant discontinuity and fragmentation of care can add to an already high disease burden (Nolte & McKee 2008) at the same time as increasing care costs through the duplication of interventions, omissions in treatment and miscommunication. Patient safety is also threatened (Boerma 2006). Whilst improvement initiatives have typically focused on optimising the clinical aspects of chronic care, this alone has not been as effective as wider initiatives that have included service redesign (Coleman *et al.* 2009, Curry & Ham 2010, Goodwin *et al.* 2012). How and where care is provided has important implications for the effectiveness and sustainability of long-term care, and strong primary care is considered to be central to improving patient outcomes and controlling costs (Roland *et al.* 2007). Patient-centred care, self-management support, improved continuity and coordination have all been identified as key contributors of quality in chronic care but can only be delivered through patients, professionals and organisations working more collaboratively together (Wagner 1996, Greaves & Campbell 2007).

Chronic kidney disease (CKD) describes abnormal kidney function and/or structure. It is common, frequently unrecognised, and it often exists together with other conditions (for example, cardiovascular disease and diabetes). The risk of developing CKD increases with age, and some conditions that coexist with CKD become more severe as kidney dysfunction advances. CKD covers a spectrum of health states including an asymptomatic period which is potentially detectable. Tests for CKD are both simple and widely available, and there is evidence that treatment can prevent or delay progression, reduce or prevent the development of complications and reduce the risk of cardiovascular disease. In cases where progression cannot be prevented, kidney function may deteriorate to stage 5, requiring life-saving dialysis, a kidney transplant or conservative management.

Estimates suggest that there about 4.5 million people in England with CKD. Since 2006, the prevalence of CKD has been reported annually in general practice and has seen a steady rise from 3% to 4.3% in 2009/10. However, compared with an estimated prevalence of 8.8%, diagnosis and ascertainment nationally is still only around half of the expected prevalence. Overall, there are an estimated 1.95 million people in England with undiagnosed CKD, who are therefore untreated and at risk of faster disease progression.

The policy context

In 2010, the UK government set out its long-term vision for the future of the National Health Service (NHS) and health services in England in the NHS White Paper, *Equity and Excellence: Liberating the NHS*. It committed to put the patient at the heart of services through greater choice and control including:

- greater shared decision making and the principle of 'no decision about me without me'
- greater choice of treatment and access to information
- a focus on personalised care that reflects individuals' health and care needs, supports carers and encourages strong joint arrangements and local partnerships

Legislation to support this policy direction has since been enacted in the Health and Social Care Act (2012). The White Paper also committed the NHS to focus on outcomes and the quality standards that deliver them. The government's objectives are to reduce mortality and morbidity, increase safety, and improve patient experience and outcomes for all. To this end, quality standards, developed by the National Institute for Health and Clinical Excellence (NICE), will inform the commissioning of all NHS care.

This approach builds upon and develops further the improvements achieved by the implementation of the National Service Frameworks (NSFs). The NSFs set clear quality requirements for care, based on the best evidence of what treatments and services work most effectively, seeking to ensure an equity of services irrespective of where they are delivered. The NSF for renal services (Department of Health 2004–05) placed a strong emphasis on identifying the condition early in primary care settings, slowing down its progress and minimising its impact on people's lives. It led to significant improvements in the way kidney disease is managed. The NICE quality standards take this further and are a set of specific, concise statements that act as markers of high-quality, cost-effective patient care, covering the treatment and prevention of different diseases and conditions. Derived from the best available evidence

Table 1.1 NHS Quality and Outcomes Framework: five domains, three dimensions.

Domain 1	Preventing people from dying prematurely	
Domain 2	Enhancing quality of life for people with long-term conditions	Effectiveness
Domain 3	Helping people to recover from episodes of ill health or following injury	
Domain 4	Ensuring people have a positive experience of care	Experience
Domain 5	Treating and caring for people in a safe environment and protecting them from avoidable harm	Safety

© The Health and Social Care Information Centre.

such as NICE guidance and other accredited sources, they are developed independently by NICE in collaboration with the NHS, social care professionals, their partners and service users. The quality standards are organised around five national outcome goals or domains, covering the breadth of NHS activity (Table 1.1), and they address the three dimensions of quality: clinical effectiveness, patient safety and patient experience. They enable:

- health and social care professionals to make decisions about care based on the latest evidence and best practice
- patients to understand what service they can expect from their health and social care providers
- NHS trusts to quickly and easily examine the clinical performance of their organisation and assess the standards of care they provide
- commissioners to be confident that the services they are providing are high quality and cost-effective

NICE published its quality standards for chronic kidney disease in 2011 (Table 1.2).

In addition to informing commissioning decisions, quality standards can also be aligned with the NHS funding system to encourage providers to follow best practice. In 2011, a best practice tariff for renal dialysis was introduced, paying significantly more for dialysis sessions that are delivered through definitive access (arteriovenous fistula or graft) than for those that are not. This is known to be better for patients because the faster flow rates result in more effective and efficient dialysis and it is much safer because of the reduced risk of infection. The level of the tariff was set so that providers with 75% (increased yearly by 5% to meet the Renal Association clinical guidelines of 85%) of their patients on definitive access would receive the same level of funding as under the previous system. In addition to rewarding services that do better than this,

Table 1.2   NICE quality standards for chronic kidney disease.

1	People with risk factors for CKD are offered testing, and people with CKD are correctly identified.
2	People with CKD who may benefit from specialist care are referred for specialist assessment in accordance with NICE guidance.
3	People with CKD have a current agreed care plan appropriate to the stage and rate of progression of CKD.
4	People with CKD are assessed for cardiovascular risk.
5	People with higher levels of proteinuria, and people with diabetes and microalbuminuria, are enabled to safely maintain their systolic blood pressure within a target range 120–129 mmHg and their diastolic blood pressure below 80 mmHg.
6	People with CKD are assessed for disease progression.
7	People with CKD who become acutely unwell have their medication reviewed, and receive an assessment of volume status and renal function.
8	People with anaemia of CKD have access to and receive anaemia treatment in accordance with NICE guidance.
9	People with progressive CKD whose eGFR is less than 20 mL/min/1.73 m², and/or who are likely to progress to established kidney failure within 12 months, receive unbiased personalised information on established kidney failure and renal replacement therapy options.
10	People with established renal failure have access to psychosocial support (which may include support with personal, family, financial, employment and/or social needs) appropriate to their circumstances.
11	People with CKD are supported to receive a pre-emptive kidney transplant before they need dialysis, if they are medically suitable.
12	People with CKD on dialysis are supported to receive a kidney transplant, if they are medically suitable.
13	People with established kidney failure start dialysis with a functioning arteriovenous fistula or peritoneal dialysis catheter in situ.
14	People on long-term dialysis receive the best possible therapy, incorporating regular and frequent application of dialysis and ideally home-based or self-care dialysis.
15	People with CKD receiving haemodialysis or training for home therapies who are eligible for transport have access to an effective and efficient transport service.

National Institute for Health and Clinical Excellence (2011) 'Chronic Kidney Disease quality standard'. London: NICE. Available from www.nice.org.uk. Reproduced with permission.

the tariff also provided a strong lever for those that were below this level to bring their services in line with best clinical guidance.

A similar tariff for multi-professional outpatient clinics encourages providers to offer patients with complex needs appointments with a multi-professional team (for example, a doctor and a psychologist or social worker) so that patients are given more choice and control and are able to move to their chosen treatment pathway more quickly. In facilitating support for patient choice and engagement as described in the White Paper, the NHS requires better systems that make it easier for different professionals and services to work more collaboratively together, providing more coordinated and seamless pathways of care. In addition to commissioning more integrated services, commissioners are also able to incentivise providers to deliver services in new ways through the Commissioning for Quality and Innovation (CQUIN) payment framework. This enables commissioners to make a percentage of payments to providers contingent on achieving locally agreed quality improvement goals.

The structure of commissioning is also changing. The Health and Social Care Act paves the way for the introduction of clinical commissioning groups (CCGs), consortia of GP practices that work together to commission services for their local populations. While some elements of kidney care, for example dialysis and transplantation, will be commissioned at a national level, CCGs will be responsible for local services to identify and manage CKD in the community. As member organisations, they will be able to engage with their member GPs on improving standards and sharing good practice; and with their population-based approach they are best placed to look at the most appropriate approaches to the prediction and prevention of CKD and proactive targeted interventions for their patients.

At the time of writing the Department of Health is consulting on a cardiovascular disease outcomes strategy. One of the main aims of this is to better integrate care across a range of associated chronic conditions including CKD, hypertension and diabetes.

The role of primary-care-based integrated teams

While there have been significant improvements in services for people with CKD in recent years, to achieve the ambitions set out in the *Equity and Excellence* White Paper and the best practice guidelines, a greater focus is needed on establishing integrated primary-care-based teams. An important role for these teams will be in determining which groups of patients can be safely managed in primary care and identifying those with more complex needs who are likely to benefit from specialist services. Most stages of CKD can be effectively managed in the community, and this is particularly so in patients whose condition is stable and who require only routine estimated glomerular filtration rate (eGFR) monitoring and lifestyle advice and support such as smoking cessation or weight management.

Appropriately trained nurses can carry out many roles in primary care that have previously been delivered by secondary care specialists. For example, the Intravenous Iron at Home initiative in Cornwall provides CKD patients with iron injections in the community or in their own home, saving them journeys of up to an hour each way for a 10-minute appointment in hospital. The service is more convenient for patients; it is safer, as there is a lower risk of developing a healthcare-acquired infection; and it saved the NHS an estimated £150 000 in 2010, based on 217 patients with an average of six appointments each year and with a third of them requiring transport or recouping travel costs.

Moving appropriate services to primary care is often cheaper and more patient-centred. Coordinating services can further improve the patient experience by avoiding duplication and omissions of care. People with CKD often have other chronic conditions and will typically receive care from a number of professionals across a number of organisations. Continuity and consistency of care can be improved by multiple providers agreeing roles and responsibilities in the patient pathway and effectively reducing 'duplicate' monitoring appointments and investigations. For example, patients frequently complain about needing to give blood tests for each clinic they attend. It would be more efficient and cost-effective and deliver a better patient experience if one blood test was taken and the results shared across the primary-care-based team. Coordination of care is dependent upon fluid data flows which ensure that patient-related information accompanies the patient to every healthcare encounter.

There are several innovative examples of primary and secondary services working together to offer patients a more joined-up and convenient service while using resources more wisely. For example, an e-mail helpline run by kidney consultants in South Tees is enabling GPs to provide timely, convenient and more efficient care for their patients with kidney disease. GPs can send e-mail questions or queries about specific patients and get a reply within a few hours. This means that patients can receive expert advice and care much more conveniently from their GP and are spared unnecessary hospital visits. The ability to offer more timely care, reduce hospital referrals and discharge patients sooner from outpatient follow-up enables a much more efficient use of NHS resources. The initiative has been well received by GPs and has helped to form strong and positive relationships between hospital consultants and their colleagues in general practice.

There is scope to greatly improve the early identification of patients with CKD. Local health needs assessments have not always been particularly effective at identifying the likely prevalence of the disease, as evidenced by the patchy estimates of the total CKD population. The government's recent introduction of 'Health Checks' in general practice has incentivised the widespread assessment of vascular risk, including CKD. Other initiatives aimed at identifying, monitoring and managing people at risk from chronic conditions are ongoing locally. The Greater Manchester Collaboration for Leadership in Applied Health Research and Care (GM-CLAHRC) is one such programme, and it has recently illustrated the potential benefits for patients with vascular conditions, including CKD, from service providers working collaboratively across traditional boundaries.

Improved assessments will also enable primary-care-based integrated teams to take more of a 'population health' approach which aims to improve the health of a population as a whole rather than narrowly focusing on those with specific conditions. Population health management (PHM) is distinguished from disease management by including more chronic conditions and diseases, by use of a single point of contact and coordination, and by predictive modelling across multiple clinical conditions. PHM is considered broader than disease management in that it also includes enhanced care management for individuals at the highest level of risk and personal health management for those at lower levels of predicted health risk. Better understanding of local population health needs will enable a reduction in the significant variation in services and outcomes across the country.

From theory to the frontline

There is a clear vision, supported by evidence and clinical guidelines, for improved and more coordinated renal services centred on primary-care-based integrated teams. But how is this being put into practice? Across the NHS there are fantastic examples of good practice and innovative ways of enabling more integrated, seamless and patient-centred care. However more needs to be done to share examples, tools and resources to enable all patients to benefit. At a systems level, there is a wide range of levers and incentives for the commissioning and provision of quality services.

The NICE quality standards set out clear criteria for commissioners of services, and the use of the CQUIN payment framework enables commissioners to reward quality improvements. The NICE quality standards and best practice guidelines such as those from the Renal Association provide a useful guide to areas of focus for improvement. Consistent data collection and sharing between providers and commissioners, through the national Renal Dataset, offers an established set of metrics on which to base assessments of performance. Similarly, the Quality and Outcomes Framework (QOF) provides a set of financial incentives for general practices to carry out certain activities which promote consistency and equity of care. Since 2006, through the QOF, GPs have been paid partly on the basis of how well they identify patients with chronic kidney disease and how well they manage their care.

In secondary care, the use of CQUIN and other financial levers, such as best practice tariffs for haemodialysis and multi-professional clinics, are incentivising best practice and discouraging avoidable variation in care. This will not only lead to improvements in the care provided, but will also have implications for how secondary care services work with primary care, driving improvements across the patients' pathways. For example, providers who are referred patients who require acute dialysis will not be able to offer this through arteriovenous fistula or graft as these can take up to six months to establish. This means that they will be unable to meet the requirements of the best practice tariff, creating a strong incentive to work closely with primary care colleagues to ensure that appropriate referrals are made in a timely manner.

Care or management plans

Early detection is essential in establishing a proactive plan of care, the aim of which is to reduce the impact of CKD on a patient's life and to minimise the risks of the patient's condition suddenly deteriorating into a crisis. This is costly both for the patient and for the health service. All people identified with CKD should be referred to an integrated vascular risk clinic and offered appropriate investigations, including renal ultrasound and immunological tests, to come to a timely diagnosis of the cause of CKD, with referrals to a nephrologist where indicated by the clinical guidelines. Care plans should be developed in partnership between the patient and the integrated team. Self-management should be encouraged and facilitated. Named providers involved in the patient's care should be listed, along with their responsibilities, and these may include nephrologists, dietitians, physiotherapists, nurse specialists, psychologists and social workers. Care planning requires the patient's participation in decision making about his or her own health and care. The aim is to make decisions informed by the best available evidence and consistent with the patient's views on what is important. This often requires ongoing discussions between healthcare professionals, the patient and the patient's family. Evidence shows that involvement in care planning improves patients' ability to self-care, improves concordance with treatment plans and improves their overall health outcomes. For patients referred to secondary care, an increased use of multi-professional clinics will encourage this to happen from the outset, and the care plan will be shared with the patient's GP and community team so that care can be continuous across different providers.

CKD encompasses a number of health states, and care plans are typically individualised to reflect this. They include information on the extent of monitoring and support patients managed in primary care will require, including triggers for when reference to the specialist team is indicated. Regular monitoring and assessment of patients with CKD in primary care reduces the risk of patients 'late presenting', which often prevents a necessary preparation process in which patients have the opportunity to discuss their treatment options over time. The care plan will also set out what other support the patient needs, for example in terms of psychological support or social care. Clinicians and patients report that care planning can also enhance clinic appointments, as less time is needed to explain test results or treatment plans. Within nephrology, partners and/or families are often involved in shaping the treatment plan as patients can become quite dependent upon them for help and support. In providing services for people with CKD it is important to include the needs of any carers involved with the patient as they can often be the sole reason that the patient can be managed at home. This is particularly true for patients on dialysis who need support with travel or with home haemodialysis, which has to be a partnership between the patient and the carer. From the carer's perspective, satisfactory involvement in care planning and decision making requires a strong sense of inclusion in the process. Additionally, carers need to feel that there is someone they can contact when they need to and that the service is responsive to their needs. Key to the achievement of a patient-centred service is the provision of better information for patients about their condition and its management. The care plan will allow patients to be offered information from a variety of sources in formats to suit their preferred learning styles. This will also include greater access to peer support networks, including peer support for carers.

Conclusion

The needs of people with chronic conditions are complex and varied, and change over time. In meeting these needs, services have traditionally been disease-specific, increasingly specialised and fragmented – factors that perpetuate service inefficiencies, rising costs and patient dissatisfaction. Recent health policy is aimed at addressing these issues by ensuring that services focus more proactively on population health and the wider determinants of health and illness. More emphasis is placed on patients being engaged in their care management, and services working more collaboratively, particularly in primary care. Central to the success of this approach is an individualised plan of care that proactively circumscribes interventions and ensures that professional and patient responsibilities are identified and information appropriately accompanies the patient.

References

Boerma, W.G.W. (2006) Coordination and integration in European primary care. In: *Primary Care in the Driver's Seat? Organizational Reform in European Primary Care* (ed. R.B. Saltman, A. Rico & W.G.W. Boerma), pp. 3-21. Open University Press, Maidenhead.

Coleman, K., Mattke, S., Perrault, P.J. & Wagner, E.H. (2009) Untangling practice redesign from disease management: how do we best care for the chronically ill? *Annual Review of Public Health*, **30**, 385-408.

Curry, N.A. & Ham, C. (2010) *Clinical and Service Integration: the Route to Improved Outcomes*. Kings Fund, London.

Department of Health (2004-05) *National Service Framework for Renal Services*. Department of Health, London.

Department of Health (2005) *Supporting People with Long Term Conditions: an NHS and Social Care Model to Support Local Innovation and Integration*. Department of Health, London.

Department of Health (2006) *Our Health, Our Care, Our Say: a New Direction for Community Care*. Cm 7881. Department of Health, London.

Department of Health (2010) *Equity and Excellence: Liberating the NHS*. The Stationery Office, London.

Department of Health (2011) Ten things you should know about long term conditions. http://www.dh.gov.uk/en/Healthcare/Longtermconditions/tenthingsyouneed toknow/index.htm (accessed September 2012).

Goodwin, N., Smith, J., Davies A., *et al.* (2012) *Integrated Care for Patients and Populations: Improving Outcomes by Working Together.* A report to the Department of Health and the NHS Future forums. Kings Fund, London.

Greaves, C.J. & Campbell, J.L. (2007) Supporting self-care in general practice. *British Journal of General Practice*, **57**, 814-21.

Health and Social Care Act (2012) http://www.legislation.gov.uk/ukpga/2012/7 (accessed September 2012).

National Institute for Health and Clinical Excellence (2011) *Chronic Kidney Disease Quality Standard.* http://www.nice.org.uk/guidance/qualitystandards/chronickidney disease/ckdqualitystandard.jsp (accessed September 2012).

Nolte, E. & McKee, M. (eds) (2008) *Caring for People with Chronic Conditions: a Health Services Perspective.* Open University Press, Maidenhead.

Roland, M., McDonald, R. & Sibbald, B. (2007) *Can Primary Care Reform Reduce Demand on Hospital Outpatient Departments?* NHS Service Delivery and Organisation, London.

Wagner, E.H., Austin, B.T. & Von Korff, M. (1996) Organizing care for patients with chronic illness. *Milbank Quarterly*, **74**, 511-44.

Resources

Department of Health Publications. http://www.dh.gov.uk/health/category/publications (accessed September 2012).

NHS Kidney Care. http://www.kidneycare.nhs.uk (accessed September 2012).

East Midlands Public Health Observatory (2009) CKD Prevalence Model. http://www.apho.org.uk/resource/item.aspx?RID=63798 (accessed September 2012).

Chapter 2
What Non-Specialists Need to Know about Chronic Kidney Disease

Graham Woodrow[1], Jeanette Denning[1] and David Lewis[2]

[1] Leeds Teaching Hospitals NHS Trust, Leeds, UK
[2] Salford Royal NHS Foundation Trust, Salford, UK

Introduction

Chronic kidney disease (CKD) is an irreversible and often progressive condition. Patients with advanced impairment of kidney function will require lifelong renal replacement therapy (RRT) by dialysis or a functioning kidney transplant to maintain survival. Patients may have CKD for a very long period of time and will become very knowledgeable and informed about their illness and the options for management. Over their lifetime many patients experience the full range of treatment options, and whilst transplantation often offers the most benefit, not all patients are suitable for this option. Advanced renal failure requiring RRT is uncommon, with 416 per million population on dialysis and 375 per million population having a functioning kidney transplant (UK Renal Registry). Thus the typical general practice will have a very small number of these patients.

Wider manifestations of CKD

Patients with advanced CKD (stage 4/5) typically have a complex medical history, suffering a variety of other coexistent serious chronic conditions. In many cases this results from their CKD being a manifestation of a condition with multiple systemic manifestations. Diabetes is the commonest and increasing cause of CKD. Many patients with advanced kidney disease due to diabetic nephropathy will have several other complications. CKD is a potent

Kidney Disease Management: A Practical Approach for the Non-Specialist Healthcare Practitioner, First Edition. Edited by Rachel Lewis and Helen Noble.
© 2013 John Wiley & Sons, Ltd. Published 2013 by John Wiley & Sons, Ltd.

risk factor for the development of cardiovascular disease, and is typically associated with hypertension, as well as being a complication of conditions such as diabetes and hypertension which are associated with increased cardiovascular disease risk. Thus ischaemic heart disease, heart failure, peripheral and cerebrovascular disease are common in patients with CKD. Patients with diabetes typically suffer the most from severe and complex vascular disease. The increasing prevalence of CKD with age means that many patients will have other chronic conditions also more common in older people. This complexity can reduce therapeutic options and challenge effective management.

Renal replacement therapy

Advanced CKD may eventually progress to the stage where remaining kidney function is not sufficient to keep the patient free of significant symptoms of kidney failure, or eventually to maintain survival. At this point replacement of kidney function by dialysis or transplantation is required. This is typically when kidney function has decreased to a glomerular filtration rate (GFR) of 10 mL/min/1.73 m^2 or less, although it should be noted that some patients are more symptomatic at a higher estimated GFR (eGFR), which is why patients should be individually assessed at regular intervals. In patients with progressive CKD, discussions and counselling to inform the patient about possible options for RRT, and to prepare for this, will begin well before this point is reached. Some patients, however, may remain free of symptoms or are undiagnosed with CKD until presenting acutely (and urgently) with advanced disease. These 'unplanned starts' or 'crash landers' often require prompt commencement of dialysis.

Options for the management at this advanced stage of kidney disease (CKD stage 5) include the different forms of dialysis, haemodialysis, peritoneal dialysis and kidney transplantation. Some patients, typically those of older age and with other chronic conditions, who have greater frailty and more limited life expectancy, may opt for a non-dialytic pathway of care. When kidney function falls to the point where dialysis is usually started, those patients who choose not to have dialysis, or are clinically unsuitable for dialysis, will commence a supportive and palliative pathway, widely referred to as conservative management or active supportive care. This decision may arise from a personal choice regarding the balance of the potential adverse impact of therapy on the patient and his or her quality of life, versus the potential extension of duration of life or improvement in symptoms that would be achieved from dialysis, which may be relatively modest in such patients.

For those following a dialytic pathway, a major consideration is the choice between peritoneal and haemodialysis as an initial mode of therapy. The majority of patients may be suitable for either form, and the final decision will be down to the individual patient in combination with education and guidance from the clinical team. Importantly, it should be explained to patients that rather than making a long-term irreversible decision, many patients will change between different dialysis modalities over their lifetimes, either for clinical reasons (including complications of the initial dialysis modality), or through patient choice for personal and lifestyle reasons. This is the idea of integrated care, whereby best use of all available therapies is made during a patient's lifetime. Kidney transplantation may provide the best outcomes in terms of survival and rehabilitation, but only a proportion of patients with advanced CKD will be suitable to be considered for transplantation. The majority of patients will receive some form of dialysis before they receive a kidney transplant. However, an increasing proportion may undergo a pre-emptive transplant before needing to start dialysis. This is most likely when there is adequate time for transplant workup before potentially needing to start dialysis, and particularly if the patient has a possible living transplant donor.

Supporting the patient at the key decision-making points of the pathway may be formalised as 'shared decision making', and it benefits from the increasing availability of tools such as patient decision aids.

Features of advanced CKD and general aspects of management

Features and complications of CKD arise from a combination of loss of excretory function which leads to accumulation of 'uraemic toxins'; loss of homeostatic regulation including fluid balance, blood pressure and acid–base regulation; and loss of endocrine effects of the kidney including reduced production of erythropoietin and vitamin D metabolism. Dialysis only partly corrects the abnormalities of stage 5 CKD. Clearances of small solutes by standard dialysis techniques are only equivalent to a small percentage of normal kidney function. Other abnormalities such as homeostatic regulation and endocrine function are only replaced partially or not at all by dialysis. Managing abnormalities of renal failure in patients on dialysis also includes important contributions from nutritional management and drug therapy.

Gastrointestinal and nutritional abnormalities

An extensive list of symptoms and complications may occur in patients with kidney failure, though symptoms may be mild or non-existent until advanced renal failure occurs. Gastrointestinal and nutritional abnormalities are important features. Loss of appetite due to uraemic toxicity, weight loss and nausea can lead to nutritional depletion, and these are often important triggers for commencing dialysis.

Nutritional management, with regular assessment and support by a renal dietitian, is an important part of the basic care of patients on dialysis (see Chapter 9). Malnutrition and wasting are common and associated with reduced patient survival. The pathogenesis is complex, with a variety of contributory factors. Intake of protein and calories is often suboptimal due to reduced appetite. This arises from a multitude of factors including the

effects of metabolites retained in renal failure on appetite, effect of multiple medications and delayed gastric emptying. In addition, multifactorial psychosocial factors result in a high incidence of anxiety and depression in this population, which are further compounded by lack of employment and financial insecurity. Dietetic management includes assessment of the adequacy of dietary intake and advice regarding alteration of diet to meet targets for nutritional intake and the use of supplements where required. Other factors leading to wasting, including catabolic processes due to uraemia and inflammation, are not reversible by increasing dietary intake. Specialist dietetic input also includes assessment and advice regarding the intake of potassium, phosphate, sodium, water and micronutrients. Complex relationships between these components of diet require expert dietetic management to avoid changes aimed at one abnormality having unintended adverse consequences (e.g. potassium or phosphate restriction leading to inadequate intake of other nutrients such as protein).

Fluid balance management

Earlier stages of CKD may result in reduced urinary concentrating ability with polyuria and sometimes a tendency to fluid depletion. When renal disease becomes more advanced a tendency to fluid retention is the norm. Fluid excess may manifest with features which are clinically indistinguishable from cardiac failure, with ankle swelling, elevated jugular venous pressure, pulmonary venous congestion or pulmonary oedema. However, the treatment of an acute presentation with standard heart failure therapy may be ineffective. Importantly fluid excess may also manifest as hypertension, even in the absence of other obvious features of fluid excess. Chronic volume overload is believed to be an important contributor to the development of cardiac dysfunction – both through the effects of hypertension and as a direct effect of volume overload. The presence of left ventricular hypertrophy or impaired function is an important adverse risk factor for reduced survival in dialysis patients.

Fluid balance management is an essential aspect of RRT. Hydration depends on a balance between fluid intake and removal. Residual kidney function and urine volume progressively decline after starting dialysis, with patients often eventually becoming anuric. Excess fluid is removed by dialysis and residual urine output, where present, may be enhanced by large doses of loop diuretics (which increase urine volume but not clearances). Patients will also have an individualised restriction of fluid intake, which may often be as low as 1000 mL/day when there is little residual kidney function. It is essential that fluid restriction is accompanied by sodium restriction, because high salt intake will result in excess thirst and difficulty in complying with fluid restriction. As hypertension may partly result from fluid status, managing elevated blood pressure will typically involve assessment by the supervising team and consideration of whether alterations of fluid management are needed in the first instance, rather than simply starting or increasing antihypertensive therapy.

Anaemia

Anaemia arises principally from reduced production of the hormone erythropoietin by the kidney. Other contributing factors include functional iron deficiency, which presents as normal iron stores determined by serum ferritin, but elevated percentage of hypochromic red blood cells on a full blood count. Management includes optimising iron status followed by treatment with an erythropoiesis-stimulating agent (ESA) or derived analogues. Iron may be administered orally but is often poorly absorbed, and side effects such as constipation may be a particular problem in patients on peritoneal dialysis. Alternatively iron is often administered intravenously, and a range of preparations are available with differing administration schedules which are well tolerated. Correction of severe anaemia by ESAs results in marked improvement in patient wellbeing. The reduced requirement for blood transfusion has a number of major benefits, including avoiding sensitisation against possible transplant donor antigens. Recent evidence suggests that complete correction of anaemia by erythropoietin rather than partial correction does not confer any benefits and may even be detrimental, particularly in those with underlying cardiovascular disease. Thus guidelines for anaemia management state target haemoglobin ranges which are less than the normal population range, and suggest that adjustment on an individual basis may be appropriate. The major hazards of ESA therapy include the development of accelerated hypertension and encephalopathy if patients are not appropriately monitored or if the rise in haemoglobin is too rapid (administration is contraindicated where blood pressure is uncontrolled). There is also an increased risk of haemodialysis vascular access thrombosis.

Bone mineral metabolism

Abnormalities of bone mineral metabolism are highly prevalent in CKD. Elevated serum phosphate results from reduced renal excretion of phosphate taken in from dietary sources. Reduced metabolism (1-alpha-hydroxylation) of vitamin D results in reduced vitamin D activity. The effects of this include a reduction in serum calcium concentrations and secondary hyperparathyroidism. Management of hyperphosphataemia includes dietary restriction and the use of medication taken at meal times, in order to bind dietary phosphate in the gastrointestinal tract and prevent its absorption. Phosphate binders include calcium compounds such as calcium carbonate or acetate, and non-calcium binders such as the organic polymer sevelamer, and lanthanum carbonate. Phosphate is also removed from the body by dialysis.

Active analogues of vitamin D such as alfacalcidol and calcitriol are used to treat hypocalcaemia and secondary hyperparathyroidism. Tertiary hyperparathyroidism may develop, where parathyroid hormone (PTH) secretion is inappropriately high, despite the development of hypercalcaemia, and this is treated by suppression of parathyroid hormone activity by the calcimimetic drug cinacalcet, or definitive surgical parathyroidectomy in patients fit for the surgery. Skeletal symptoms may result from hyperparathyroid bone disease or an osteomalacia picture, and some patients may develop adynamic bone disease (often from therapeutic over-suppression of PTH secretion). Other clinical features include itching, which may be associated with hyperphosphataemia and may have a significant effect on quality of life in dialysis patients. An important change of emphasis in managing these abnormalities has resulted from the increasing evidence of disturbed bone mineral metabolism and vascular calcification and the relationship of accelerated cardiovascular disease.

Life expectancy in CKD

Life expectancy is significantly reduced in patients with advanced CKD. The data show the median remaining life expectancy for dialysis patients to be 20 years for patients in the 25-29-year-old age group, and 4 years for those aged over 75 years (UK Renal Registry 2010). The major cause of increased mortality is accelerated cardiovascular disease, with a range of underlying risk factors. Traditional cardiovascular risk factors remain important. Hypertension is common, of long duration and often severe. Control of hypercholesterolaemia improves cardiovascular outcomes in non-dialysis CKD patients with lesser degrees of renal impairment. The evidence in dialysis patients is less conclusive. The pathophysiology of cardiovascular disease in CKD differs from the population without renal disease, with predominant features including medial vascular calcification and left ventricular hypertrophy and dysfunction, rather than the typical arterial atheroma seen in non-renal patients. Specific risk factors in renal failure may include the effects of volume overload, vascular calcification, anaemia, an inflammatory state and increased oxidative stress, which are common in advanced CKD.

Management of drug therapy

Management of medication in patients with advanced CKD is complex because of the effects of renal disease and dialysis on drug pharmacokinetics, and the potential for interactions with the often extensive lists of prescribed medications (see Chapter 8). Many drugs require dose reduction or cannot be used in patients with advanced renal failure or on dialysis, because of the risk of accumulation and toxicity resulting from reduced renal excretion. Commonly used drugs where there is a need for marked dose reduction and a risk of serious toxicity include digoxin and antivirals such as aciclovir. Many antimicrobials also require dose reduction. It is essential when prescribing any drug for these patients to be aware of recommendations for prescribing regimes in renal disease. Metformin should be used with caution in renal impairment and is contraindicated in the presence of a GFR less than 30 mL/min/1.73 m^2 because of the risk of life-threatening lactic acidosis. Nephrotoxic drugs should still be avoided in dialysis patients who have residual kidney function.

The wider multidisciplinary team

Management of patients with stage 5 CKD in secondary care involves an extensive multidisciplinary team, including doctors, specialist nurses, pharmacists, dietitians, psychologists and social workers. Close links exist with a range of other secondary care specialties including radiology, vascular surgery, general and transplant surgery, diabetes and cardiology. When these patients present to other specialties or primary care, early liaison with the renal team may be needed to facilitate investigation (for instance limitations on the use of radiological contrast or to interpret blood results) and management. This includes situations where illness may relate to CKD or its treatment such as dialysis- or transplant-related sepsis, fluid overload and hypertension or electrolyte abnormalities, or where advice regarding drug therapy may be required. Discussion with the specialist team is also required where hospital admission is necessary, either for planning provision of dialysis during the patient's illness or admission, or for advice regarding care of a kidney transplant.

Urea and creatinine

Serum urea and creatinine levels remain markedly elevated in dialysis patients compared with patients with normal kidney function. Values are strongly influenced by dietary protein intake or muscle mass respectively and are not a useful measure of the efficacy of dialysis, which is determined by measurements of clearance by the dialysis procedure. Relatively lower serum urea and creatinine values are actually associated with worse outcomes on dialysis, often reflecting poor nutrition or wasting rather than more efficient dialysis.

Haemodialysis

Haemodialysis involves circulation of blood from a patient through an extracorporeal circuit during a dialysis treatment session. Blood passes through hollow fibres made of a semipermeable material, which separates the blood from dialysate solution flowing outside the fibres. Haemodialysis replaces the excretory function of the kidney by diffusion of substances from a patient's blood to the dialysis fluid, which then goes to waste. The dialysis process also corrects acidosis by diffusion of bicarbonate from the dialysis fluid into the patient's blood. Excess fluid is removed during the dialysis process through ultrafiltration achieved by a hydrostatic pressure difference applied across the dialysis membrane. Haemodialysis may take place as an outpatient in a central hospital haemodialysis unit, in a satellite unit (more stable patients dialysed away from main unit setting, with lower levels of on-site medical supervision, and usually closer to home) or in the patient's home. Typical haemodialysis treatments last four hours and are performed three times per week (though there may be some variation tailored to the individual patient requirements). Most units offer two or three dialysis shifts a day - morning, afternoon and sometimes evening - and patients are usually offered a Monday, Wednesday, Friday or Tuesday, Thursday, Saturday schedule. In both timetables there is a two-day gap, which is associated with increased morbidity and mortality, and patients have to be extra-careful regarding their fluid and dietary intake. Haemodialysis at home allows the possibility of more frequent and/or longer dialysis treatments. This may result in less variation in fluid and biochemical state between treatment sessions, or a greater degree of clearance. An increasing, but typically small, proportion of haemodialysis patients actually perform their dialysis at home following appropriate training, experiencing clinical benefits, greater flexibility of daily activities and better rehabilitation compared with hospital-based treatment.

Managing dry weight

Fluid gained since the last treatment will be removed during haemodialysis to return the patient to his or her 'dry' weight – the weight at which a patient is believed to be at the optimum state of hydration. Weight gain between the end of one haemodialysis session and the start of the next is ascribed to fluid taken in by the patient between dialysis sessions, and not lost through any residual urine output or insensible loss, and will be removed by dialysis. Dry weight needs to be adjusted over time to account for changing nutritional state and underlying normal 'flesh weight'. Excessive fluid intake results in increasing fluid overload and hypertension with their associated effects prior to the next dialysis session. The need to remove large volumes of fluid during a haemodialysis treatment is likely to accentuate the adverse symptoms associated with dialysis.

Vascular access

Vascular access is one of the most critical aspects of haemodialysis. This is the route via which blood is removed and returned to the patient's circulation. The optimal form of vascular access is an arteriovenous fistula. This involves surgical formation of an anastomosis between an artery and vein (e.g. radiocephalic or brachiocephalic anastomoses) which results in a high flow of arterial blood being diverted into the vein, which subsequently develops into the fistula. Over a period of time the vein becomes dilated and the walls thicken with a high blood flow, making it suitable for repeated punctures by needles at the start of dialysis. A mature fistula facilitates the movement of blood through the dialyser at the desired flow rates (typically 300 mL/minute). The advantages of fistulae over other forms of vascular access include greater access survival and lowest risk of infection and thus subsequent bacteraemia or septicaemia. Ideally formation of a fistula should take place at least 2–3 months before the start of haemodialysis is anticipated so that it has time to mature.

If a patient requires haemodialysis when there is no working fistula (e.g. if the patient presents too late or the fistula has not matured), haemodialysis may take place through a catheter inserted into a central vein, usually jugular or if inappropriate a femoral vein. Disadvantages of this means of access include an increased risk of sepsis, poorer blood flow rates and thus efficiency of dialysis, and usually limited access survival due to development of infection or occlusion by thrombus. Finding suitable sites for the formation of an arteriovenous fistula may become increasingly difficult, from progressive loss of sites of previous failed access, central venous stenosis from previous catheters, damage to peripheral veins from cannulae or phlebotomy, or intrinsically poor-calibre vessels. Where formation of a fistula is impossible, an arteriovenous graft made of artificial material may be inserted between an artery and vein. These lie subcutaneously and can be needled like an arteriovenous fistula. However, the greater risk of thrombosis or infection and subsequent failure due to the presence of foreign material makes these less desirable than native arteriovenous fistulae. Difficulties in obtaining vascular access in some patients can reach a potentially life-threatening stage, due to a practical inability to perform further life-preserving haemodialysis. Thus preservation of veins that may be required for future access is of critical importance in patients with potentially progressive or advanced kidney disease. Ideally phlebotomy or insertion of intravenous cannulae should avoid the forearm and preferably be carried out in the dorsum of the hand, or if necessary in the antecubital fossa. In a patient with a fistula (or graft), it is essential that the arm is not used for measuring blood pressure, phlebotomy or the insertion of intravenous cannulae. If a patient notes that the normal thrill (or bruit) they can feel on palpating the fistula disappears, they should contact their unit urgently for treatment. This may include anticoagulation with intravenous heparin and surgical or radiological intervention to restore the patency of the fistula. Other complications of fistula formation include distal ischaemia resulting from a 'steal' syndrome, and arm swelling due to venous hypertension.

The dialysis procedure

The haemodialysis procedure typically requires administration of intravenous unfractionated or low-molecular-weight heparin to prevent blood clotting in the dialysis circuit. Alternative strategies may be employed in patients where this would be associated with a risk of haemorrhage. During the dialysis procedure, there is a major change in blood biochemistry and significant volumes of fluid are typically removed, typically 1–2 litres. In some patients the haemodynamic impact of haemodialysis induces hypotension and the patient feels ill during the procedure. Despite the improvement in blood biochemistry and fluid status derived from a haemodialysis treatment, patients typically feel less well immediately afterwards, and patients may take up to six hours following the procedure to fully recover. Intolerance of the haemodialysis procedure is most likely to occur in patients who are frail and have cardiac disease.

Hyperkalaemia

Hyperkalaemia is an important complication of renal disease due to reduced excretion of ingested dietary potassium, and it can result in potentially fatal cardiac arrhythmias without prior warning symptoms. Some experienced patients are aware of high potassium levels due to a tingling sensation. Potassium is removed during the haemodialysis procedure. This means that serum potassium will progressively increase between dialysis sessions in patients with little remaining kidney function. Control of dietary intake of potassium is required to prevent dangerously high blood levels prior to the following dialysis session. Serum potassium will be particularly low when measured immediately after a haemodialysis session because of the removal of potassium from the extracellular space, and will then rise significantly over the following few hours due to redistribution from potassium within cells (which accounts for 98% of total body potassium). This means that a low serum potassium immediately after haemodialysis may be misleading and should not be corrected by potassium replacement, as it will spontaneously rise shortly afterwards. Potassium is present in the dialysis fluid in haemodialysis to prevent serum potassium falling too low during dialysis. In contrast, the continuous nature of peritoneal dialysis results in a more steady serum concentration of potassium.

Peritoneal dialysis

Peritoneal dialysis (PD) works on the principle that dialysis fluid is infused into the peritoneal cavity, and dialysis occurs by movement of substances between the patient's blood, flowing in the capillaries in the peritoneal membrane lining the peritoneal cavity and organs, and the dialysis fluid. Thus the capillaries act as the 'dialysing membrane', As with haemodialysis, in PD substances to be removed diffuse from the patient's blood into the dialysis solution, and acidosis is corrected by the diffusion of a buffer substance (either lactate or bicarbonate) from the dialysis fluid into the patient. Unlike haemodialysis, PD achieves fluid removal by the osmotic effect of the dialysis solution. Most peritoneal dialysis solutions contain high concentrations of glucose, which exert an osmotic effect, allowing fluid to be removed from the patient (rather than the dialysis fluid being absorbed from the peritoneal cavity). Different glucose-concentration solutions are available to allow individualised dialysis prescription according to the amount of fluid that needs to be removed from a particular patient, and the function of the peritoneal membrane (which varies between patients). A significant amount of glucose may be absorbed by the patient from the dialysis solution. This can lead to effects including transient hyperglycaemia (or alteration in glycaemic control in patients with diabetes) and contributes to lipid abnormalities and some weight gain.

The peritoneal catheter

Access to the peritoneal cavity is via a PD catheter, which may be inserted under local or general anaesthetic. The catheter is inserted in the midline in the lower abdomen below the umbilicus, and is tunnelled laterally to emerge from one side of the lower abdominal wall. Care of the catheter, with appropriate cleansing and dressing of the exit site and immobilisation of the catheter, is important to reduce the risk of infections and aid healing. It is essential that access to the peritoneal cavity is by correct protocol and sterile technique to reduce the risk of microbial contamination. It will require the use of the appropriate dialysis equipment, which may preclude sampling of dialysis fluid in a patient presenting as an emergency to another hospital which does not have a PD unit unless the patient or carer is able to provide the equipment and perform the procedure themselves. Similarly, in patients unable to care for the catheter themselves or in situations where infection is suspected, liaison with the specialist team will ensure that appropriate advice and support is provided.

PD procedures

PD is a home-based therapy, usually performed by patients themselves. Important features of PD are greater freedom from hospital attendance and the schedules of haemodialysis and greater flexibility. This may particularly suit patients who are working, and may provide a greater opportunity for travel and holidays. PD nurses have a major role in the management, including training patients in the techniques of dialysis, follow-up and support both in hospital and in the community, monitoring and adjustment of treatment, and identifying and managing complications.

There are two main forms of PD: continuous ambulatory peritoneal dialysis (CAPD) and automated peritoneal dialysis (APD). CAPD involves manual exchanges of bags of dialysate. The standard volume is 2 litres but this may be adjusted up or down depending on the patient's size and tolerance. When a patient performs a CAPD exchange, fluid that has been present in the peritoneal cavity for a period typically of 4–6 hours drains by gravity into a bag temporarily attached to the catheter, the bag and fluid are then discarded as waste, and fresh dialysate is drained in. This will remain in situ (whilst the patient is performing his or her usual daytime activities, or is asleep overnight) until the next exchange. Typically a patient on CAPD will perform four exchanges spaced out during the day, every day, and each exchange will typically take up to 30 minutes. The bags of fluid are heated by an electric warmer prior to infusion. Dialysis fluid is present continuously except during the short period when the spent fluid is drained out and fresh fluid is about to drain in at each exchange. Exchanges can be performed at home or in any suitable enclosed area.

APD occurs at night when the patient is in bed. The patient attaches the PD catheter to an APD cycling machine which automatically drains dialysis fluid in and out of the patient several times overnight during sleep. At the end of the programme, a volume of fluid remains in the patient and the machine is disconnected.

The choice between CAPD and APD is largely down to patient choice. Some patients prefer the simpler CAPD method, whereas others find overnight PD frees them from multiple daytime procedures and suits their lifestyle and routine better. In some patients, the permeability of their peritoneal membrane may subsequently mean that one particular form of PD is better suited to providing optimal removal of solutes or fluid. The characteristics of the patient's peritoneal membrane can be measured.

Whilst most PD patients perform their own dialysis exchanges, a number may rely on a helper, often a family member, to perform part or all of the dialysis procedures. In this situation, APD may often be the preferred mode of PD, requiring fewer procedures to be performed during the day. Assisted PD is a recent service provision in some areas, referring to dialysis performed by a nurse or healthcare worker in the community, where patients are unable to do it themselves. Generally APD requires the patient or carer to connect the catheter to the machine and to disconnect following completion, although assisted CAPD is possible with adequate available nursing assistance (with extensive experience of this described in France).

Fluid balance management in PD patients

Fluid balance management is an important aspect in PD, and is key to optimising patient outcomes. As in haemodialysis, fluid retention results in hypertension and cardiovascular disease. Altering fluid status in a PD patient may involve adjustments to the dialysis prescription, modification of salt and fluid intake, an assessment of residual function and the possible use of high-dose loop diuretics (under the supervision of the multidisciplinary team). Some patients will benefit from the use of an alternative solution containing a high-molecular-weight glucose polymer called icodextrin for one of their exchanges per day. This is particularly effective in removing fluid when the dialysate dwell is for longer periods of time (e.g. during the day for APD and overnight for CAPD). Small amounts of circulating oligosaccharides such as maltose are derived from this solution, and may impact on some diagnostic assays. In particular, this can lead to overestimation of capillary blood glucose by some glucometers utilising the glucose dehydrogenase–pyrroloquinoline quinone (GHD-PQQ) measurement system. Consequently, there can be a risk of undiagnosed hypoglycaemia due to incorrectly high glucose readings and it is essential that PD patients using this dialysis solution, who require capillary glucose monitoring, are issued with a suitable glucometer, and that if they are hospitalised, measurements are made with an appropriate system. Falsely low serum amylase measurements may also occur, making this an unreliable test to exclude acute pancreatitis in patients using this solution.

Infection and peritonitis

The major modality-specific complications of PD relate to infection. The catheter exit site, where the catheter emerges from the abdominal wall, may become infected. This often responds to a course of antibiotics and will typically require at least two weeks of antibiotic therapy. In cases where the infection is persistent or recurrent, it is usually necessary to remove the catheter and a insert new catheter to allow ongoing PD. A number of different protocols are used to care for the PD catheter to reduce the chances of infection. Exit-site infections are commonly due to *Staphylococcus aureus* or *Pseudomonas aeruginosa*. NICE guidelines (2011) recommend that patients should undergo prophylactic therapy against infection (particularly *Staphylococcus aureus*) with a range of regimes, typically including nasal or exit-site application of mupirocin. Patients are trained to recognise and report features suggestive of infection and will undergo regular assessment by specialist PD nurses.

PD peritonitis is a serious complication in which infection occurs in the peritoneal cavity. It may arise from contamination at the time of performing PD connections, spread of infection from an exit-site infection, or infection with enteric organisms arising from translocation or bowel pathology. Infections may range in severity from the development of cloudy dialysate with minor abdominal pain only, to severe infections with severe pain and peritonism, development of ileus and systemic manifestations of sepsis. Patient education and training in PD includes a major focus on aseptic technique to reduce the risk of infection. Guidelines suggest that an incidence of peritonitis of less than one episode every 18 patient months should be achieved by PD programmes, and with careful attention to factors affecting the risk of peritonitis significantly better rates can be achieved. Peritonitis often resolves with appropriate antibiotic therapy. A range of regimes, often including intraperitoneal administration of antibiotics, is used according to local unit protocols derived in combination with local microbiology advice.

A significant proportion of peritoneal infections do not resolve and require removal of the PD catheter and a transfer to haemodialysis. In this situation a small proportion of patients may subsequently return to PD, but even with successful treatment of infection, recurrent PD peritonitis may lead to long-term loss of peritoneal membrane function and failure of PD. In some episodes, peritonitis may be very severe and potentially life-threatening.

Diagnosis of PD peritonitis involves inspection of drained dialysate and measurement of fluid white cell count, with a count of >100 white cells/mm^3, with more than 50% comprising polymorphs, being diagnostic. Fluid is then cultured (with specific sample collection and processing protocols to maximise the likelihood of a positive culture) to determine the causative organism and antibiotic sensitivity. **It is important that any PD patient with abdominal discomfort or cloudy dialysate is seen urgently in a PD unit to allow appropriate assessment and diagnostic tests**. Delay can lead to major deterioration and worse outcomes. If a PD patient presents acutely with abdominal symptoms to a hospital that does not have a renal unit, urgent contact should be made with the supervising renal unit for advice about further investigation and management, and the need for urgent transfer.

Other causes of abdominal pain

A variety of other causes exist for abdominal pain in PD patients. Constipation is a common feature in PD and is very important to prevent, as it can lead to poor fluid drainage, catheter migration within the peritoneal cavity (on an abdominal x-ray the tip of the catheter should lie well into the pelvic cavity) and loss of function. PD patients are typically prescribed regular laxatives, even in the absence of constipation. Pain may result from infusion of the dialysis fluid (with many dialysis fluids having an acidic pH). Patients on PD may also suffer the same conditions that cause abdominal pain in non-PD patients. Thus the possibility of acute abdominal conditions (diverticulitis, acute pancreatitis, biliary disease, visceral perforation, acute appendicitis, gynaecological disease etc.) should also be considered in the PD patient presenting with abdominal pain and features of 'PD peritonitis'.

Maintenance of residual renal function

Residual kidney function, even in patients receiving dialysis, is an important contributor to fluid management and small solute clearances and a positive determinant of patient survival. The preservation of residual kidney function should be encouraged by avoiding dehydration and nephrotoxic agents such as non-steroidal anti-inflammatory drugs (NSAIDs). Although PD allows for a more liberal fluid and dietary intake, most patients typically still require some fluid restriction.

Other complications of PD

Effective dialysis in PD requires the free flow of fluid in and out of the peritoneal cavity. Common causes of impaired drainage include constipation and malposition of the peritoneal catheter within the peritoneal cavity. In both cases large doses of laxatives are often effective, with increased bowel activity sometimes helping a catheter to move back into a position where function is restored. Occlusion due to fibrin may be resolved by infusing heparin into the catheter. With persistent non-function of the catheter, and other causes such as occlusion by omentum, surgical replacement or repositioning of the catheter may be required.

Mechanical complications can arise from the effect of raised intra-abdominal pressure due to the presence of the dialysis fluid. Hernias are a common complication in PD and usually require surgical repair. Fluid leaks may also occur subcutaneously, leading to abdominal wall swelling, or into the pleural cavity, leading to a pleural effusion (a diagnostic pleural aspiration will indicate low levels of protein and high levels of glucose). A swollen scrotum may also indicate a leak. Leakage of fluid may occur externally around the catheter exit site. This is most common early after catheter insertion and may require temporary rest from PD to allow healing. Because of the difference in intra-abdominal pressure when patients are recumbent, those with complications relating to the pressure associated with CAPD may be effectively treated with smaller volumes on APD overnight and the peritoneal cavity left empty during the day when the patient is ambulant. This approach may allow continuation of PD, until surgical repair if required or resolution of a leak, rather than switching to haemodialysis, and also facilitates early resumption of PD after surgical repair of hernias unless particularly large or complicated. Some patients on PD may also have sufficient residual kidney function to be able to hold off from dialysis for a short period of time, rather than having to undergo temporary haemodialysis, in cases where PD therapy needs to be interrupted.

In a proportion of patients the effectiveness of PD will diminish. This may occur acutely, for example after severe or non-resolving peritonitis, or more gradually from prolonged exposure to PD dialysis fluid. The reduction in dialysis and fluid removal may require a switch to haemodialysis.

A rare but serious complication that may occur in patients after several years on PD is encapsulating peritoneal sclerosis (EPS). A thickened and inflamed peritoneal membrane leads to cocooning of the patient's intestines, resulting in bowel obstruction and malnutrition. This often presents when the patient is no longer receiving PD, after transfer to haemodialysis or renal transplantation. Optimal nutritional support and advances in surgical management in expert centres has greatly improved the outcome in this condition.

Kidney transplantation

Kidney transplantation provides the best option for rehabilitation and survival for suitable patients with stage 5 CKD. Options for transplantation include deceased donor kidneys allocated via national matching schemes and living donation. The criteria for living donation have expanded with schemes for desensitising patients who have high antibody levels against a potential donor or a different ABO blood type. In recent years altruistic donors have come forward to donate despite having no relationship to the recipient. There is also the option for multiple organ transplantation, most commonly combined kidney and pancreas transplantation for patients with stage 5 CKD and type 1 diabetes.

The transplanted kidney is usually placed in the iliac fossa, in the extraperitoneal space, with vascular anastomoses to the iliac vessels and the donor ureter to the patient's bladder. Following kidney transplantation, a patient will receive long-term immunosuppressive treatment, which is essential to prevent rejection of the kidney by the recipient's immune system. A range of immunosuppressant drugs and combinations are used. Many, but not all, patients may receive longer-term glucocorticoid therapy as part of their immunosuppressant therapy.

Assessment for kidney transplantation

All patients with stage 5 CKD should be assessed for kidney transplantation. However, contraindications are frequent such that only a proportion of patients will be deemed suitable after a detailed assessment. The most frequent cause of exclusion from transplantation is cardiovascular disease. This may result in too high a risk of surgery or too short a life expectancy for transplantation to be considered. Peripheral vascular disease may preclude transplantation because of difficulty in vascular anastomosis to diseased iliac vessels or the risk of precipitating critical distal lower limb ischaemia. Patients at high risk of or known to have cardiovascular disease will undergo extensive investigations. These typically include non-invasive assessment for cardiac function and ischaemia, with coronary angiography not uncommonly required, and imaging of pelvic and distal lower limb vessels. Obesity increases the difficulty and risks of transplant surgery and is a frequent contraindication. Sources of chronic sepsis (e.g. diabetic foot problems or chronic urosepsis associated with urological disease) need to be resolved before transplantation can be considered because of the risk of severe sepsis developing as a result of immunosuppression. A history of malignancy is also a contraindication to transplantation unless an adequate time has passed since the treatment such that the risk of developing metastatic disease is sufficiently reduced. This is to avoid transplanting a patient where residual disease may result in a short life expectancy and progression of malignant disease could be accelerated by immunosuppressive therapy. Bladder function and anatomy must be adequate. On rare occasions bladder augmentation or formation of an ileal conduit may be required before transplant listing.

Management of the kidney transplant patient

Initial transplant function may vary between patients, but in the majority will be less than the normal range of GFR, equivalent to CKD stages 3–5. Consequently, all patients with a kidney transplant should be considered to have a degree of CKD. This means that, as in non-transplant CKD patients, tight blood pressure control is an important aspect of management to slow down any further deterioration of function. Care with drug use and dosing, and avoidance of potentially nephrotoxic drugs such as NSAIDs, is important. Kidney transplant patients may also suffer the same metabolic complications of impaired kidney function as those with native-kidney CKD, including hyperkalaemia, acidosis, abnormal bone biochemistry and anaemia. Maintenance of hydration during hospital admission or acute inter-current illness is important.

Immunosuppression

Maintaining immunosuppression is a crucial consideration in managing a patient with a kidney transplant. Even a short interruption to treatment can precipitate an acute rejection episode. It is essential that patients do not miss their therapy in situations where oral intake is impaired. In some cases such as fasting for surgery it may still be possible to take medication orally. Where this is not possible, including in patients with severe acute gastrointestinal dysfunction, immunosuppressant drugs must be administered intravenously, with accurate dose adjustment. Care should be taken when transplant patients are admitted to a hospital ward, not routinely stocking these drugs, to ensure a supply is made available. Patients will often have their own supply in the interim. Patients on long-term steroid therapy must continue to receive this during inter-current illnesses. If necessary steroids may be administered intravenously and the dosage increased to cover the stress of acute illness.

Immunosuppressant drugs have a number of critical interactions with commonly prescribed drugs. Calcineurin inhibitors (ciclosporin and tacrolimus) have relatively narrow therapeutic ranges, with high concentrations resulting in adverse effects including serious nephrotoxicity, whereas inadequate concentrations may result in the risk of damage or loss of the transplant from acute rejections. A number of medications may cause a marked increase in the levels of these agents, including erythromycin, clarithromycin and diltiazem. Low levels may result from enzyme-inducing agents including rifampicin, phenytoin and carbamazepine. However, the list of drugs potentially interacting is extensive, and it is important to check for potential interactions of any new drugs prescribed to transplant patients. The prescription of allopurinol can result in dangerous potentiation of the effects of azathioprine in patients receiving this immunosuppressant drug, with the risk of severe bone marrow suppression, and it is contraindicated except under expert supervision with major dose reduction and very careful monitoring. The availability of alternative immunosuppressant agents such as mycophenolate mofetil means that immunosuppressant regimes may more often be changed to facilitate management of gout in patients with a kidney transplant. Acute gout poses a difficulty as well due to contraindication to NSAIDs, with other agents such as colchicine, or a short course or increased dose of corticosteroids, usually being used.

As the major immunosuppressant drugs have come out of patent restrictions, bio-similar medications have been developed. These may offer financial advantages but there are risks if the various versions of a drug are considered interchangeable where blood levels and bioavailability may be different. It is recommended that a patient is maintained on a single brand of these medicines, and that any changes are managed under specialist supervision.

Infection after renal transplantation

Infection is one of the major complications following renal transplantation. A transplant patient with features of infection requires urgent assessment because of the possibility of severe or unusual underlying causes. Common bacterial infections may be more common or severe as a result of immunosuppression, and because of reduced immunity patients are also susceptible to opportunistic infections with atypical organisms. Urinary infection is common, due to abnormal urinary tract anatomy, and can result in severe sepsis. Varicella zoster may manifest as shingles in patients with a history of chickenpox. Exposure to the virus in patients without immunity from previous infections may result in overwhelming zoster infection. Patients are advised to avoid contact with individuals with active disease, and if they do have contact they require urgent testing for immunity and administration of zoster immunoglobulin if not immune. Antiviral prophylaxis may be prescribed for a period following transplantation when the risk of clinic infection is believed to be highest. Cytomegalovirus infection may result from transfer of the virus from the transplant kidney or reactivation of the virus present in the patient from prior infection. This can lead to severe illness with features including fever, pneumonitis, colitis, retinitis, hepatitis, leucopenia and thrombocytopenia. Other opportunist infections that may occur following transplantation include *Pneumocystis jirovecii* pneumonia, *Candida* infections and tuberculosis. BK virus infection is an important cause of renal transplant dysfunction.

Acute transplant dysfunction

There are a number of causes of reduced function in a kidney transplant. This requires urgent specialist investigation including imaging and potentially a biopsy, and management to reduce the possibility of longer-term irreversible reduction of function and shortened survival of the transplanted kidney, or even acute loss in some cases. Causes of acute transplant dysfunction include acute rejection, urine infection, calcineurin inhibitor nephrotoxicity, obstruction and transplant vascular complications. It should be remembered that relatively small increments in serum creatinine from a baseline in or near the normal range may represent a significant reduction in actual GFR. Recurrence of some underlying causes of the patient's original kidney failure, particularly certain types of glomerular disease, may occur in a kidney transplant, in some cases leading to significant loss of function.

Other complications of kidney transplantation

Following kidney transplantation patients are subject to an increased risk of a number of complications. Cardiovascular disease remains a major cause of morbidity and mortality. Hypertension is common following kidney transplantation, and dyslipidaemia is common. The majority of transplant patients will have a degree of impairment in kidney function compared with healthy individuals and so are subject to the increase in cardiovascular risk associated with CKD. New-onset diabetes may develop following kidney transplantation, with causal factors including the effects of some immunosuppressant drugs such as tacrolimus, ciclosporin and corticosteroids, and weight gain due to improved appetite and a more liberal diet following transplantation.

Immunosuppression leads to an increased risk of malignancy. This is most marked for skin malignancy – particularly squamous cell carcinoma. Patients are counselled after transplantation to use high-factor sun blocks and avoid excess sun exposure. Any new skin lesions in a transplant patient require a low threshold for referral for expert dermatological assessment. Regular cervical smear screening is important in women. Rare malignancies, including a range of lymphoproliferative disorders, may also occur. Patients receiving long-term steroid therapy may develop complications including osteoporosis. Management of this may include regular monitoring by bone densitometry, but the situation is complicated by the coincident presence of metabolic bone disease due to previous and ongoing reduced GFR.

Over time there may be gradual decline in kidney function such that eventually patients may return to a level of stage 5 CKD and the need for commencement of dialysis and/or further transplantation. There is a range of contributing causes to chronic allograft nephropathy, including immuno-logical and non-immmunological factors, such as hypertension and calci-neurin inhibitor toxicity. With increasing numbers of patients undergoing transplantation, transplant failure makes up an increasing proportion of patients starting dialysis. As well as issues of psychological adjustment there are other differences to new-start patients. These include risks of infection of haemodialysis or peritoneal dialysis access and the tapering off of immunosuppression. This is undertaken slowly enough to avoid an acute rejection episode of the otherwise failed graft. These patients are likely to have higher levels of immune sensitisation, and to have a longer wait for another transplant.

As transplant immunosuppression has evolved, one-year graft survival has improved, although long-term outcomes have not reflected this. The best marker for long-term graft survival is kidney function a year after transplant. One-year graft survival is over 90% in the UK, and at five years it is over 80%.

Conclusion

As the population of people with CKD and other chronic conditions increases, so too will their management in non-specialist areas. This chapter illustrates the main technical and practical aspects of renal replacement therapy, including transplantation. It discusses some of the common clinical issues associated with treatment modalities and how these may be optimally managed.

References and resources

Department of Health (2004) *National Service Framework for Renal Services. Part One:Dialysis and Transplantation*. Department of Health, London. http://www.dh.gov.uk/en/Publicationsandstatistics/Publications/PublicationsPolicyAndGuidance/DH_4070359 (accessed September 2012).

Dudley, C., Bright, R., & Harden, P. (2011) Assessment of the potential kidney transplant recipient. Renal Association. http://www.renal.org/ClinicalGuidelinesSection/AssessmentforRenalTransplantation.aspx (accessed September 2012).

Farrington, K., & Warwick, G. (2009) Planning, initiating and withdrawal of renal replacement therapy. Renal Association. http://www.renal.org/clinical/guidelinessection/RenalReplacementTherapy.aspx (accessed September 2012).

National Institute for Health and Clinical Excellence (2011) Preparing for renal replacement therapy. http://www.nice.org.uk/guidance/qualitystandards/chronickidneydisease/preparingforrenalreplacementtherapy.jsp (accessed September 2012).

UK Renal Registry (2010) 13th Annual Report 2010. http://www.renalreg.com/Reports/2010.html (accessed September 2012).

Chapter 3

A Practical Approach to Chronic Kidney Disease in Primary Care

Hugh Rayner[1], Rajib Pal[2] and Indranil Dasgupta[1]

[1]Heart of England NHS Foundation Trust, Birmingham, UK
[2]General Practitioner, Birmingham, UK

Introduction

In the past, kidney medicine was regarded as rare, complicated and best left to the specialists. Now it is an everyday part of primary care. This chapter demystifies chronic kidney disease. It uses real-life examples and gives practical suggestions for treating patients with chronic kidney disease (CKD) from stages 1 to 5. Citing recent trial evidence, it signposts you to information and educational resources for clinicians and patients.

Joined-up working – the key to success

Good primary care, working in collaboration with secondary care, is crucial for the successful management of all stages of CKD (defined below). To confirm CKD, estimated glomerular filtration rate (eGFR) must be measured on two or more occasions at least three months apart. Most patients with CKD are at stage 3 and can be managed effectively in the community. Specialist care is more often needed for stages 4 and 5 (Table 3.1).

CKD that has worsened over years can suddenly decompensate to cause acute problems such as pulmonary oedema. If you identify such patients early, you will reduce the chances of an emergency hospital admission. Following an unplanned start of dialysis, mortality in the first year is doubled and time spent in hospital tripled compared to a planned start. Thanks to improved collaborative working, the proportion of patients starting dialysis without adequate pre-dialysis nephrology care has fallen steadily in the UK (Figure 3.1).

Kidney Disease Management: A Practical Approach for the Non-Specialist Healthcare Practitioner, First Edition. Edited by Rachel Lewis and Helen Noble.
© 2013 John Wiley & Sons, Ltd. Published 2013 by John Wiley & Sons, Ltd.

Table 3.1 Definitions of the KDOQI (National Kidney Foundation Kidney Disease Outcomes Quality Initiative) stages of chronic kidney disease.

Stage	eGFR (mL/min/1.73 m²)	Description
1	90+	Normal kidney function but urine findings or structural abnormalities or genetic trait point to kidney disease
2	60–89	Mildly reduced kidney function and other findings point to kidney disease as for stage 1
3A	45–59	Moderately reduced kidney function
3B	30–44	Moderately reduced kidney function
4	15–29	Severely reduced kidney function
5	<15 or on dialysis	Very severe or end-stage kidney failure

National Institute for Health and Clinical Excellence (2011) 'CG 73 Chronic Kidney Disease: early identification and management of chronic kidney disease in adults in primary and secondary care'. London: NICE. Available from www.nice.org.uk/guidance/CG73 Reproduced with permission. Accurate at time of going to press.

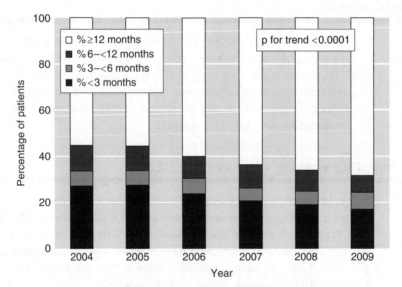

Figure 3.1 The lengths of time patients were known to a kidney unit before the start of renal replacement therapy (RRT), as a percentage of all patients starting. Data are from 11 English kidney units that have reported data continuously since 2004 with >75% data completeness. 6730 patients started RRT in the UK in 2009. (2010 Report, Nephron Clinical Practice Vol. 119, Suppl. 2, 2011, UK Renal Registry 2010, 13th Annual Report of the Renal Association, Caskey F, Dawnay A, Farrington K, Feest T, Fogarty D, Inward C, Tomson CRV, UK Renal Registry, Bristol, UK. The data reported here have been supplied by the UK Renal Registry of the Renal Association. The interpretation and reporting of these data are the responsibility of the authors and in no way should be seen as an official policy or interpretation of the UK Renal Registry or the Renal Association).

Should I screen for CKD?

Screening of the well population for albuminuria or eGFR is not cost-effective, nor clinically appropriate. On the other hand, targeted screening is worthwhile. The National Institute for Health and Clinical Excellence (NICE) recommends that you offer testing for CKD, i.e. blood for eGFR and urine for albumin : creatinine ratio (ACR), to people who have:

- diabetes, hypertension, ischaemic heart disease, heart failure, peripheral vascular disease or cerebrovascular disease
- structural urinary tract disease, kidney stones or an enlarged prostate
- a multisystem disease with potential kidney involvement (for example, systemic lupus erythematosus)
- a family history of stage 5 CKD or hereditary kidney disease
- blood or protein detected on urinalysis

Test for microscopic haematuria with reagent strips; there is no need to use urine microscopy to confirm a positive result. Confirm results of 1+ or more by a positive result on two out of three repeat tests. Investigate for urinary tract malignancy in appropriate patients, such as those aged over 50 years. Macroscopic haematuria always requires an explanation, whatever the age of the patient.

Patients with persistent microscopic haematuria who do not have proteinuria or a known urological cause are still at an increased risk of hypertension, proteinuria and reduced GFR in the future. They should be followed up annually with repeat testing for haematuria and proteinuria on urinalysis, GFR and blood pressure, as long as the haematuria persists.

NICE recommends that people receiving long-term lithium have their eGFR checked at least every six months, and those taking systemic non-steroidal anti-inflammatory drugs (NSAIDs) at least annually.

Should I tell patients they have CKD?

The term 'chronic kidney disease' includes two words that mean different things to patients and clinicians. To lay people, 'chronic' implies severe, serious, and possibly cancer; and 'disease' relates to feeling ill. None of these applies to the early stages of CKD, and it is important not to raise unnecessary alarm. However, no one wants to miss the opportunity of avoiding severe illness in the future.

When explaining CKD, you may find it helpful to use an everyday analogy - money. 'At birth, your two kidneys normally have enough kidney function to last your whole life. This is like having a lot of money in your kidney savings account. As you get older, your kidney function slowly goes down and your savings are used up. If you do not have normal kidneys to start with, or they lose function more quickly than normal, you will run out of "savings" and start to feel ill.'

How do I identify patients who are likely to be troubled by their kidney disease?

Simple urinalysis is the first step. The greater the amount of proteinuria or albuminuria, the greater is the risk that GFR will decline in future. Conversely, the absence of albuminuria in a patient with CKD is a good prognostic sign.

Patients who suffer one or more episodes of acute kidney injury (AKI, previously termed acute renal failure) have an increased risk of advanced CKD and death in the long term, even if their GFR recovers following the acute episode. Highlight this past medical history in the patient's records.

Younger patients with kidney disease, such as damage due to reflux in childhood, are at a high lifetime risk of progressing to advanced CKD. They may develop proteinuria and hypertension before the decline in eGFR. Similarly, patients under the age of 40 years with idiopathic hypertension are at a higher risk, especially if they have proteinuria.

You should counsel younger women with CKD or proteinuria about their increased risk of complications during pregnancy. The lower the eGFR, the more likely they are to have pre-eclampsia, premature delivery and neonatal complications. In turn, the increased kidney blood flow in pregnancy can accelerate the decline in GFR. Advise women about contraception and consider referring them to an obstetrician or nephrologist when they are planning a pregnancy.

Which patients should I refer to a nephrologist?

Patients without diabetes mellitus who have more than 1g per day of proteinuria (urine albumin : creatinine ratio (ACR) >70 mg/mmol or protein : creatinine ratio >100 mg/mmol) are likely to have a significant glomerular disease. You should refer them for consideration of a renal biopsy.

In patients with diabetes, these levels of proteinuria put them at very high risk of progressive loss of GFR. They too should be referred to a nephrologist to make sure everything is being done to reduce this risk.

Patients with both haematuria and proteinuria (urine ACR >30 mg/mmol with dipstick haematuria) who do not have symptoms of urinary tract infection may have glomerulonephritis. This may be a kidney-limited disease with no other symptoms, or it may be part of a systemic disease such as systemic lupus erythematosus (SLE) or vasculitis. A vasculitic illness may include low-grade fever, tiredness, weight loss, joint pains, rash and ENT symptoms. GFR may decline rapidly, so repeat the eGFR measurement a week after the first detection. Discuss the details with a nephrologist at an early stage. By getting treatment started quickly, you may avoid the need for long-term dialysis.

Patients with poorly controlled blood pressure (>150/90 mmHg) have a higher risk of kidney failure and death. You may need specialist advice in a minority of patients whose blood pressure is not controlled even though they take the medication regularly.

Older men with reduced eGFR and symptoms such as frequency, dribbling and nocturia may have chronic urinary retention and hydronephrosis. These men may be unaware of the severity of the problem, assuming the symptoms are a sign of old age. If you find suprapubic dullness and a palpable bladder you should make an urgent hospital referral. Otherwise request an ultrasound scan to be performed within four weeks.

Patients with stage 4 CKD who are not unwell and whose eGFR is not deteriorating may not need to attend an outpatient appointment. However, it is a good idea to get the advice of your local nephrologist to make sure nothing important is being overlooked. Conversely, patients with stage 5 CKD should be reviewed in person by a nephrologist so that a long-term treatment plan can be discussed, unless they are too unwell or unwilling to travel to the clinic (see Chapter 10).

You may be asked to monitor patients with uncommon causes of CKD as part of a disease-specific management plan. This should include clear criteria for when to seek advice from the nephrologist. All patients with CKD should take an active part in their care plan, monitoring their own blood pressure and keeping track of their eGFR. Patients can access their own blood results securely via the internet using Renal PatientView (www.renalpatientview.org). Patients with rare kidney diseases may wish to join a self-help group linked to Rare Disease UK (www.raredisease.org.uk).

Monitoring kidney function – the power of the eGFR graph

Having identified who is at risk of kidney failure, you and the patient need a simple and effective tool for monitoring kidney function. This is the eGFR graph.

Symptoms are of no help in tracking the early stages of CKD. Instead, the eGFR graph acts as a map of the kidney history. The examples shown in Figures 3.2–3.7 demonstrate its value in describing the natural history of

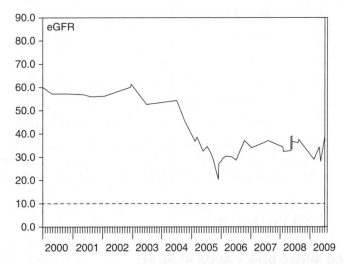

Figure 3.2 This man was referred to a nephrologist in late 2005 because of a progressive decline in eGFR. He had diabetes and was feeling more tired but did not volunteer any new symptoms. On examination, he had a prominently distended bladder. eGFR improved following catheterisation to relieve his chronic urinary retention and bilateral hydronephrosis, but sadly not to its previous level.

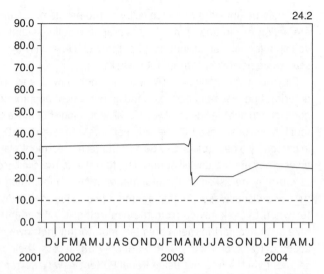

Figure 3.3 This woman had diabetes and macroscopic haematuria. An ultrasound scan revealed a renal cell carcinoma that was removed in April 2003. After the operation, her eGFR fell by 50% but then recovered slightly as some nephrons increased their filtration rate to compensate for the loss of one kidney.

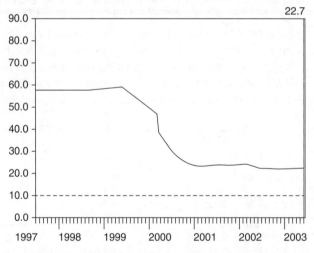

Figure 3.4 This man had peripheral vascular disease. An ultrasound scan in 2001 showed a small left kidney that had become ischaemic over the preceding two years, leading to a decline in the combined GFR of both kidneys.

kidney disease. See if you can work out from the graphs when the management could have been better.

Making sense of variation in eGFR

NICE guidance suggests that a decline in eGFR of >5 mL/min/1.73 m² per year or >10 mL/min/1.73 m² within five years should prompt a search for remediable

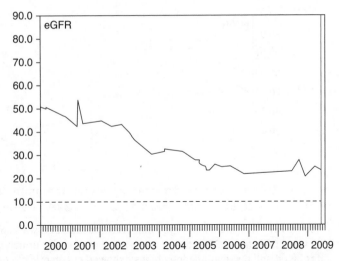

Figure 3.5 This lady had diabetes and poorly controlled blood pressure despite taking an ACE inhibitor. At her first consultation with a nephrologist in 2005, she was shown her eGFR graph and encouraged to measure her own blood pressure at home, with a target systolic pressure of less than 140 mmHg. A diuretic was added to the ACE inhibitor. Following control of her blood pressure, the decline in her eGFR was arrested.

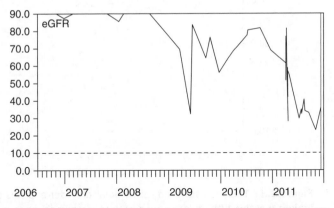

Figure 3.6 This woman had diabetes and normal kidney function until she suffered a myocardial infarction (MI) in 2009. This was complicated by acute kidney injury (AKI), which only partially resolved. In 2011 she suffered a second MI, again complicated by AKI. She was left with moderate to severe CKD and at risk of needing dialysis in the future.

causes. These numerical rules are hard to apply when the eGFR is varying month by month. The eGFR graph makes it easy to see whether a drop is part of a consistent downward trend, as in the example shown in Figure 3.8.

Judge the most recent result against the previous range of variation in eGFR for that patient. Variation is greatest when the eGFR is >60 mL/min/1.73 m². eGFR values at this level are calculated from near-normal levels of serum creatinine. Variation at lower levels of serum creatinine leads to large variation in the

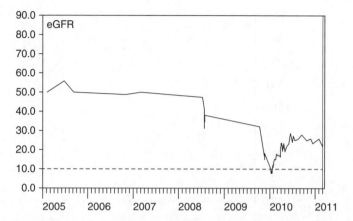

Figure 3.7 This man had type 1 diabetes and his eGFR was slowly declining. In late 2009, his eGFR dropped much more rapidly and urinalysis was positive for blood and protein. A kidney biopsy showed crescentic glomerulonephritis. His GFR responded well to high-dose steroids and cyclophosphamide.

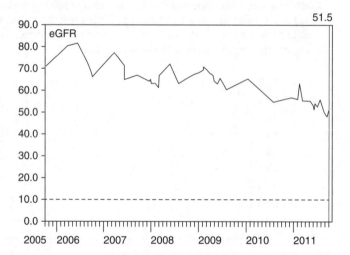

Figure 3.8 This man suffered with bipolar disorder and was taking long-term lithium therapy. Lithium can cause both reversible changes in fluid balance and irreversible damage to renal tubules. Reviewing the results over six years makes the declining trend due to irreversible damage obvious.

eGFR because the two are inversely related. Conversely, variations in eGFR below 45 mL/min/1.73 m^2 are more likely to represent important changes in GFR.

Misleading estimates of GFR

Estimated GFR (eGFR) is calculated from the serum creatinine concentration. Changes in the serum creatinine concentration may not always be due to changes in the true GFR.

Variation in the laboratory creatinine assay is proportionally greatest in or near the normal range. Hence most laboratories do not report an exact figure for eGFR >60 mL/min/1.73 m² because the confidence interval at this level is so wide.

Changes in meat intake can lead to small short-term changes in the serum creatinine concentration. However, you do not usually need to ask the patient to starve before the blood test.

Body builders and athletes have a large muscle mass. This produces a lot of creatinine, increases the serum creatinine level and gives a misleadingly low eGFR. In addition, some take dietary protein and creatine supplements. These are digested to release urea and creatinine into the bloodstream and so further reduce the estimated GFR. To give a more consistent estimate of GFR, take blood samples after a week without supplements.

Take care to use the eGFR correction factor for African-Caribbean race where appropriate – this increases the estimate by 21%.

Some drugs can alter the serum creatinine level without affecting the true GFR. Trimethoprim inhibits the secretion of creatinine by the kidney tubules, leading to a rise in serum creatinine concentration. Fibrates can alter muscle creatinine metabolism and increase serum creatinine. As the true GFR is unaltered, these effects do not alter the serum urea – a helpful pointer to this explanation.

Finally, if a change in eGFR seems inexplicable, check whether the patient's gender has changed between male and female, either surgically or inadvertently on the blood test request form.

If you suspect that a persistently reduced eGFR may not reflect the true GFR, check for other signs of kidney disease such as proteinuria, hypertension and abnormalities on ultrasound.

What does proteinuria mean?

Proteinuria results from damage to the endothelial cells and basement membranes of the glomeruli. It is also a sign of damage to the vascular endothelium elsewhere in the body. Hence, proteinuria is an important risk marker for future worsening of kidney function and for cardiovascular events such as myocardial infarction and stroke. The greater the amount of proteinuria, the greater is the risk of loss of GFR and the faster it is likely to decline.

Day-to-day variation in the amount of proteinuria can be large, 100% or more, due to the effects of exercise, diet and blood pressure. However, longer-term trends in the amount of proteinuria are useful guides to changes in the risk of kidney damage. In patients with CKD and high blood pressure, a sustained reduction in proteinuria is an encouraging sign that improved control of blood pressure is giving long-term benefits.

The strength of the correlation between proteinuria and the risk of kidney failure has led to it being used as a surrogate outcome in drug trials of patients with CKD. Unfortunately, not all ways of reducing proteinuria also reduce the risk of kidney failure. Combining drugs that inhibit the renin-angiotensin system (such as ACE inhibitors, angiotensin receptor blockers and renin inhibitors) reduces proteinuria, but longer-term trials have shown an increase in the risk of kidney failure in some patients.

Proteinuria is a guide to the long-term risk of kidney and cardiovascular disease, so there is little value in measuring it repeatedly in elderly patients with limited life expectancy.

Management of patients with CKD

Your two main roles in the management of patients with kidney disease are: (1) to minimise the cardiovascular risk associated with CKD, and (2) to reduce the rate of loss of kidney function. The actions required for both are similar. Complex management of kidney diseases, such as with immunosuppressive drugs, should remain in secondary care.

The CKD Quality and Outcomes Framework (QOF) encourages practices to develop a CKD register of patients with stage 3–5 disease, record blood pressure and urine ACR measurements at least annually, control blood pressure (target <140/85) and use angiotensin converting enzyme inhibitors (ACE inhibitors) or angiotensin receptor blockers (ARBs) in patients with proteinuria. You may wish to expand your QOF CKD register to include patients with abnormal kidneys or albuminuria and eGFR >60 mL/min/1.73 m^2.

Most patients with CKD are on at least one other chronic disease register, such as diabetes, coronary heart disease or hypertension. You may wish to operate a combined vascular disease clinic to avoid duplication of effort. Organise primary and secondary prevention of cardiovascular disease according to the usual guidelines. Most patients will need to be reviewed every 6–12 months depending on their clinical need.

Get the results of tests for serum urea and electrolytes, eGFR, corrected calcium, phosphate, HbA1c if diabetic, lipids, full blood count, and urine ACR (preferably an early-morning sample) and share them with the patient a week or two before the clinical review. During the face-to-face consultation, discuss the test results and home blood pressure readings, and agree goals for the future. Carry out a general health check, and assess any lower urinary tract symptoms and cardio-respiratory symptoms such as breathlessness and swelling.

Blood pressure – the number one priority

Effective blood pressure control is the top priority in CKD. For patients without diabetes, NICE recommends a systolic BP in the range 120–139 mmHg and diastolic BP <90 mmHg. In those with diabetes or significant proteinuria (urine ACR >70 mg/mmol), systolic BP should be in the range 120–129 mmHg and diastolic BP <80 mmHg.

Emphasise ways that the patient can take control of his or her own blood pressure. Home blood pressure meters are inexpensive. Most arm cuff meters have been validated as accurate, but wrist meters do not give reliable readings. In our experience, patients do not become anxious from measuring their own blood pressure. They may become insistent that their blood pressure is not adequately controlled, but that is to be welcomed.

Even though few doctors wear white coats, the 'white coat' effect can be very marked and lead to inappropriate escalation of medication. Home readings are a much better guide to long-term outcomes. Set a simple blood pressure goal: 'The top number should be less than 140 almost every time you check it.'

Patients often ask about possible dietary changes that may lower blood pressure. There is strong evidence that reducing daily salt intake increases the antihypertensive effect of drugs such as ACE inhibitors. In patients with CKD, lower salt intake is associated with a lower risk of CKD stage 5 (Vegter et al. 2012). Patients should not add salt at the table and should avoid processed foods with a high salt content. Salt substitutes may contain large amounts of potassium chloride, which is contraindicated in some CKD patients.

Advise patients to reduce their salt intake over a period of weeks. A rapid and large reduction will mean food suddenly tastes bland and your advice will probably be ignored. Reduce slowly and the taste buds will adapt to the new diet and food will continue to be enjoyable. Indeed, a variety of subtle flavours will emerge when the overwhelming taste of salt is removed.

Patients with CKD and hypertension lose the usual night-time 'dip' in blood pressure. Advise them to take at least one of the blood pressure agents at bedtime to maximise the blood pressure-lowering effect during sleep. Simply changing the time the tablets are taken can reduce the risk of cardiovascular events by two-thirds (Hermida et al. 2011).

Apart from blood pressure control, there is no convincing evidence to support other interventions for slowing the decline in GFR. Low-protein diet was studied in the Modification of Diet in Renal Disease (MDRD) study. The MDRD eGFR formula was the main product of this study – a low-protein diet did not have a significant effect. Similarly, lowering cholesterol does not slow the rate of decline in GFR.

Healthy living, healthy kidneys

Lifestyle advice for people with CKD is no different to general healthy living advice: stop smoking, drink alcohol in moderation and not every day, eat more fruit and vegetables, take regular exercise and, if obese, lose weight.

Smoking is a risk factor for the development CKD and is associated with more rapid decline in GFR and increased mortality. Knowledge that the kidneys are affected may help motivate a patient to quit. Signpost patients to smoking cessation support at every review.

Excess alcohol consumption contributes to CKD through its link with obesity and cardiac disease. Incorporate brief intervention, including an alcohol screening questionnaire such as the AUDIT-C, into the review.

Drinking two or more cola drinks per day, diet or regular, has been associated with a doubling of the risk of CKD. Other carbonated drinks showed no association. This may be due to the phosphoric acid in cola.

Many fruits and vegetables have an important acid-neutralising effect. If taken in sufficient amounts, they are as effective as sodium bicarbonate tablets in reducing urinary albumin excretion and other markers of kidney injury (Goraya et al. 2012).

Thirty minutes of moderately intense physical activity should be taken on a regular basis, ideally five times a week. Kidney disease is not worsened by exercise, and the health benefits of exercise extend even to patients on dialysis. Some kidney dialysis units offer exercise programmes that patients can do during the dialysis treatment.

Obesity has mixed associations with kidney disease and outcomes. It leads to increased proteinuria, and extreme obesity can cause glomerular damage (focal segmental glomerulosclerosis). On the other hand, in patients with CKD stage 5, obesity loses its association with mortality. This is possibly because it protects against malnutrition in patients with severe chronic disease.

How can I use ACE inhibitors and ARBs safely?

Drugs that inhibit the renin–angiotensin–aldosterone system (RAAS) are used frequently in patients with CKD. They include angiotensin converting enzyme inhibitors (ACE inhibitors, drug names ending in -pril), angiotensin II receptor blockers (ARBs, drug names ending in -sartan) and renin inhibitors, all of which act to reduce the effect of angiotensin II (A-II). A-II is a potent vasoconstrictor that also stimulates the adrenal glands to produce aldosterone. Aldosterone stimulates potassium excretion by the kidney tubules and is blocked by drugs such as spironolactone.

If you use them appropriately, ACE inhibitors and ARBs can protect kidney function and reduce the risks of heart failure and mortality; use them inappropriately and they can cause acute kidney injury, severe hyperkalaemia and precipitate dialysis. How can you get the balance right?

To understand how these drugs can heal and harm, you need to understand how A-II affects the kidney. A-II acts on the small muscular blood vessels that take blood away from the glomeruli (the efferent arterioles). Vasoconstriction of these vessels is needed to maintain pressure in the blood vessels behind them, i.e. within the glomeruli. This hydrostatic pressure forces fluid through the pores in the endothelial cells and across the glomerular basement membrane; in other words, it causes glomerular filtration.

Imagine you are using a garden hose on a summer's day, spraying your flowerbeds and anybody nearby. To get a strong spray you need the tap turned full

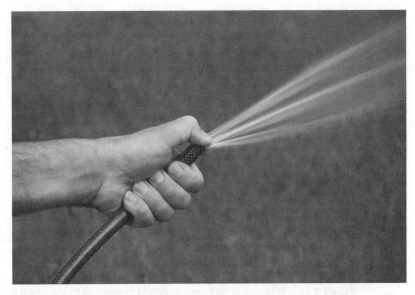

Figure 3.9 The hosepipe analogy for glomerular filtration. Glomerular filtration requires high pressure in the glomerular capillaries. Constriction of the arteriole leaving the glomerulus is like pressing your thumb on a hose. Resistance to flow out of the hose increases the pressure and creates the spray.

on. This is like a high arterial blood pressure. To vary the spray you change the resistance on the end of the hose. The harder you press with your thumb, the greater the resistance, the higher the pressure and the further the spray goes (Figure 3.9). This is like varying the resistance in the efferent arterioles – vaso-constriction increases glomerular filtration.

So if you block A-II with an ACE inhibitor, you allow vasodilatation of the efferent arterioles and relieve the pressure within the glomeruli. If this pressure was damaging the glomerular cells and membranes, reducing the pressure will reduce the damage and preserve kidney function in the long term. Proteinuria is a sign of membrane damage, and so ACE inhibitors are particularly suitable for hypertensive patients with proteinuria. Figure 3.10 shows an example of how effective an ACE inhibitor can be.

Reducing the pressure within the glomeruli can cause a drop in GFR. This may recover towards the previous level over subsequent weeks but sometimes the drop is greater and does not recover. To understand why this happens, let's return to our garden hose. If the tap attached to the hose is turned down, the spray becomes less powerful. This is like having a lower systemic arterial pressure due to cardiac failure, vasodilator drugs or salt and water depletion by diuretics or diarrhoea. If someone stands on the hose, the spray becomes even weaker. This is like narrowing the main renal arteries or the smaller arteries within the kidney, which reduces the pressure in the glomeruli. Glomerular filtration then becomes critically dependent upon there being a lot

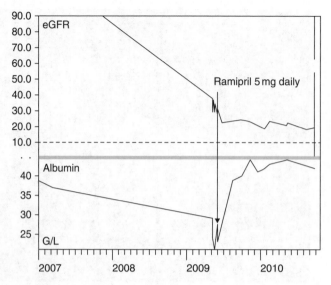

Figure 3.10 This man with type 1 diabetes presented to the renal clinic in May 2009 with gross peripheral oedema, proteinuria 10 g/24 hours and serum albumin 21 g/L, i.e. nephrotic syndrome. His eGFR had dropped from 114 mL/min/1.73 m² in March 2007 to 38 mL/min/1.73 m² in May 2009. His blood pressure was poorly controlled by a calcium channel blocker and he had not been taking an ACE inhibitor. A renal biopsy confirmed diabetic nephropathy. Ramipril 5 mg per day was started. Proteinuria reduced to <3.5 g/24 hours, oedema cleared, serum albumin returned to normal and the rate of decline in eGFR was greatly reduced.

of resistance to blood flowing out of the glomeruli. If you stop pressing hard with your thumb, the spray drops to a trickle.

Patients at risk of harm from ACE inhibitors and ARBs are those with low blood pressure due to cardiac failure and those with vascular disease who have narrowing in the renal arteries or afferent arterioles. If the eGFR drops by >25%, the ACE inhibitor or ARB should be stopped and the eGFR rechecked after 1–2 weeks.

A critical ACE inhibitor or ARB effect can be identified from the pattern of changes in serum potassium, urea and creatinine. Aldosterone normally increases potassium excretion into the urine. When it is blocked, serum potassium rises, often to >6 mmol/L. With the drop in GFR, urea increases to a greater extent than creatinine, perhaps doubling compared to a 50% rise in creatinine. This is because urea diffuses back into the bloodstream from the filtered fluid within the tubules. Creatinine cannot diffuse back and is actively pumped out by the tubules, so its rise is comparatively smaller than that of urea.

Patients who initially tolerate an ACE inhibitor or ARB may, after years of taking them, develop the distinctive abnormalities in serum potassium, urea and creatinine, as illustrated in Figure 3.11.

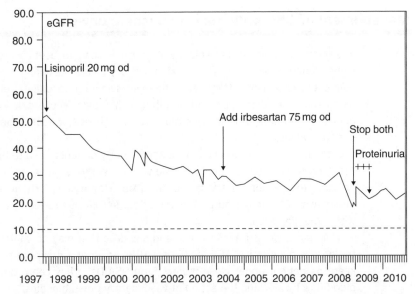

Figure 3.11 This man with diabetes was treated for many years with the ACE inhibitor lisinopril. Because his home blood pressure remained too high and eGFR was falling, irbesartan (an ARB) was added in 2004. (N.B. This preceded evidence that combination therapy can be harmful.) In 2008 there was sudden drop in eGFR, with a rise in urea to 22 mmol/L and potassium to 7.5 mmol/L. The ARB and ACE inhibitor were stopped. Potassium returned to normal and the eGFR rose towards the previous baseline. Blood pressure was controlled with other drugs. Proteinuria appeared for the first time, presumably due to increased pressure within the glomeruli.

Systematic care of the CKD population

Many patients fail to get access to treatments that would reduce their risk of kidney damage. Those who have the biggest problems with managing their own health and in accessing health care are also at the highest risk of kidney failure. This is particularly an issue with CKD because it is asymptomatic. However, patients at high risk of kidney failure can be identified from their eGFR and ACR results in existing computer databases.

Having sought these patients out, refer them to a specialist clinic at the earliest signs of progressive damage, such as heavy proteinuria or declining eGFR. Personalised education and support for self-care can then reduce their risk of progressing to CKD stage 5 (Rayner *et al*. 2011). Such organised systems can be operated within a general practice or from a hospital laboratory and kidney unit.

General practitioners, practice nurses, hospital and community-based diabetes nurses and doctors can be integrated using information technology. Shared electronic patient records can increase the efficiency and effectiveness of care. In Bradford, the number of traditional nephrology referrals has been halved, improving the lives of patients who no longer have to attend the hospital (Stoves *et al*. 2010).

Management of CKD patients who become unwell

Inter-current illness in patients with CKD may lead to acute worsening of kidney function ('acute-on-chronic kidney injury'). Patients taking diuretics are vulnerable, especially if they have high fever, sweating, vasodilatation and low blood pressure. Diarrhoea and vomiting can rapidly cause salt and water depletion. Patients with an ileostomy are at high risk of acute kidney injury due to fluid loss.

Community nurses monitoring frail and elderly patients need to be alert to these risks and seek a medical review at an early stage. A drop in blood pressure to 'low-normal' levels (e.g. 110/60 mmHg) in an elderly hypertensive person with CKD may lead to a marked drop in GFR due to reduced pressure within the glomeruli.

If the blood pressure is low, suspend any drug that may be contributing to the drop (e.g. diuretics, ACE inhibitors, ARBs or other antihypertensives) and keep the patient under close review. Stop NSAIDs – they can reduce kidney blood flow by blocking the action of vasodilatory prostaglandins.

Stop metformin in patients with diabetes if the eGFR falls below 30 mL/min/1.73 m². Metformin is not nephrotoxic and does not affect eGFR. However, it increases the risk of lactic acidosis in patients with acute kidney injury.

Once the acute illness has resolved, review the patient's medication and restart drugs when appropriate. Blood sugar control is often much worse when metformin is stopped, so restart it once the eGFR is above 30 mL/min/1.73 m². If you omit diuretics and ACE inhibitors/ARBs for too long in patients with heart failure they may slip into pulmonary oedema.

Management of patients with CKD stages 4 and 5

When the eGFR falls below 30 mL/min/1.73 m², complications of CKD become more common. These include acidosis, anaemia, falling serum calcium, and rising serum phosphate and parathyroid hormone.

Acidosis is diagnosed by serum bicarbonate <22 mmol/L. If this persists despite a diet high in fruit and vegetables, give sodium bicarbonate supplements to correct the serum level. The risk of sodium overload with these supplements is low. Correction of acidosis delays the progression of advanced CKD and the need for dialysis.

Renal anaemia can be treated with iron and erythropoietin. Do not fully correct the haemoglobin (Hb) concentration with erythropoietin as this increases the risk of stroke. Treatment is not usually started until the Hb falls below 10 g/dL. Treating anaemia does not slow down the decline in GFR.

Damaged kidneys are unable to activate vitamin D, and this leads to a fall in serum calcium. Correct this with alfacalcidol or calcitriol as these forms of vitamin D are already activated. Over-treatment may cause hypercalcaemia, leading to an acute drop in GFR. Chronic moderate over-treatment may accelerate vascular calcification. Delay treatment until the serum calcium is near or below the lower limit of normal unless there are clear signs of osteomalacia such as a raised alkaline phosphatase level. A rise in serum phosphate probably signifies advanced kidney failure and should be managed in collaboration with a nephrologist.

At least a year before the predicted time when dialysis will be needed, care should be shared with a specialist multidisciplinary 'pre-dialysis' clinic. Shared decision making is at the heart of care for patients in this clinic. Whilst a clinician can describe the symptoms and limitations likely to confront a patient, only the patient can decide how to cope with them and what adjustments to make to his or her way of life. Patient autonomy is paramount, even if the course of action the patient chooses may seem unreasonable to you.

Patients are given a choice of type of dialysis and are guided through the decision process. Informed patient choice requires information to be provided in a balanced and understandable way, clarifying how each treatment may help or hinder the patient in achieving the things that are most important to him or her. For most patients, retaining their independence is a high priority and so they are encouraged and supported in overcoming the hurdles of dialysing at home. Information for patients is available (e.g. www.patient.co.uk/health/Chronic-Kidney-Disease.htm) and NHS shared decision aids can be incorporated into the discussions (www.nhsdirect.nhs.uk/DecisionAids.aspx).

Symptoms of kidney failure such as lethargy, sleep disturbance, itching, nausea and vomiting become more severe when eGFR falls below 10 mL/min/1.73 m^2. Dialysis can safely be delayed until symptoms of kidney failure justify the burden of treatment. There is no benefit from starting dialysis earlier based upon the eGFR alone.

Long-term outcomes are much better if patients start dialysis with a permanent modality such as continuous ambulatory peritoneal dialysis (CAPD) or haemodialysis (HD) via an arteriovenous fistula. The high risk of morbidity and mortality associated with referral to a nephrologist less than three months before starting dialysis is largely due to the temporary vascular catheters needed for dialysis.

Older patients with CKD

CKD affects more than a third of those aged 75 years and over. The majority will not be aware they have a kidney 'disease' unless you tell them. Many will never be troubled directly by kidney disease. This raises the dilemma of whether you should inform elderly patients and risk causing anxiety and stress without any clear benefit.

Risk factors for progression in the elderly are proteinuria, hypertension and cardiovascular comorbidity. The decline in eGFR tends to be slower, and older patients at stage 3 with none of these risk factors are unlikely to progress to stage 5. When discussing test results, it is reasonable not to emphasise the 'chronic' and 'disease' aspects of their CKD.

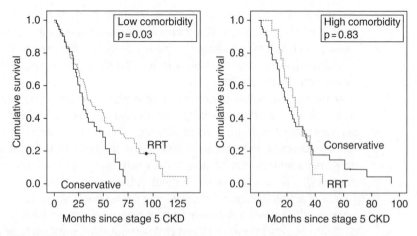

Figure 3.12 Comparison of Kaplan–Meier survival curves by modality (renal replacement therapy RRT versus conservative kidney management) in patients >75 years of age (Chandna *et al.* 2011 by permission of Oxford University Press).

The risk of complications due to CKD (such as anaemia and hyperparathyroidism) is still present in the elderly, but your response to this should be proportionate to the patient's health and life expectancy. Conversely, you may recommend treatment of systolic blood pressure >160 mmHg in people aged ≥80 years who are otherwise well (e.g. with indapamide SR 1.5 mg ± perindopril 2 or 4 mg to achieve BP 150/80), as it can reduce mortality, stroke and heart failure within a year or two of being started (Beckett *et al.* 2008).

Elderly patients with progressive stage 5 CKD do not always benefit from dialysis (Dasgupta & Rayner 2009). Those with multiple comorbidities such as ischaemic heart disease, peripheral vascular disease, diabetes, poor intellectual capacity, functional dependence and low serum albumin have a very high mortality rate on dialysis. Their quality of life often gets worse when dialysis is started. Any prolongation of life is offset by the time they spend having and recovering from the treatments. Many such patients regret starting dialysis.

Conservative kidney management is a positive alternative treatment to dialysis for such frail elderly patients. All symptomatic treatment is offered other than dialysis itself, avoiding inessential and unpalatable medications. You can refer a patient to the nephrology service specifically for such a care package to be arranged in partnership with your team.

Figure 3.12 shows two graphs from a report by the kidney unit in Stevenage, showing the survival of two groups of patients aged >75 years treated with either dialysis (renal replacement therapy, RRT; *n* = 689) or conservative kidney management (*n* = 155).

Patients with low comorbidity survived significantly longer with dialysis than with conservative care from two years after reaching stage 5 CKD. However, for some patients, quality rather than quantity of life may be much more relevant to the decision about whether or not to start dialysis.

Patients with high comorbidity survived slightly longer with dialysis during the first three years of follow-up. However, all who had dialysis died within four years of reaching stage 5. Conversely, one in five patients with high comorbidity who received conservative kidney management had much longer survival.

These figures may be helpful when you are discussing treatment options with frail elderly patients and their families. It is very difficult to predict which patients are the ones likely to survive longer without dialysis.

As part of the conservative kidney management plan, you can play an important role in coordinating services, in improving continuity of care delivered by practice nurses, district nurses, community matrons and social workers, and in linking closely with the specialist team.

When patients with end-stage kidney disease reach the terminal stage of their illness, they should have access to appropriate palliative care, which is discussed in Chapter 10.

Patients with a kidney transplant

Patients who have had a kidney transplant must remain under follow-up in secondary care. However, they will inevitably present to you, and some familiarity with common issues that affect them is useful.

Immunosuppressive drugs must be taken throughout the life of the transplant. The immune response is most suppressed during the first year after transplantation. Have a low threshold for contacting the specialist unit during this time, as the infection may be atypical and worsen rapidly. Infections of the respiratory and urinary tracts are not uncommon. The likely organism should guide your choice of antibiotic. Trimethoprim may lead to a rise in serum creatinine and hence a drop in eGFR, as explained above. This can cause uncertainty about possible transplant rejection.

Immunosuppressive drugs should be initiated in secondary care. Once the patient is stable, you may accept responsibility for prescribing them under an Effective Shared Care Agreement. The nephrologist will provide advice and monitor efficacy, side effects and drug levels. Many immunosuppressive drugs are now 'off patent' and available in a variety of generic formulations. These can have differing bioavailabilities, so it is important not to switch preparations without close monitoring by the specialist unit.

Include medications prescribed in secondary care on the patient's electronic record so that potential interactions are flagged up. You may need to alert the nephrologist about conditions that might interfere with drug absorption, e.g. diarrhoea and vomiting.

Joint pain is common in transplant patients. Avoid prescribing NSAIDs because of their potential nephrotoxicity. When treating gout, do not start allopurinol in patients taking the immunosuppressant drug azathioprine. Allopurinol blocks the breakdown of the active metabolite of azathioprine (mercaptopurine), which can lead to potentially fatal bone marrow suppression and low white blood-cell count.

As a result of long-term immunosuppression, transplant patients have an increased risk of cancer. The commonest site is the skin, and you should encourage pale-skinned patients to wear a hat and use sunscreen, even when it is not sunny. The risk of lymphoma is also increased. This can present with weight loss, sweats, sickness, abdominal pain and altered bowel habit. Other cancers are slightly more common, and so it is worth reminding women to attend for regular breast and cervical cancer screening.

Conclusions

This chapter aims to give you the essential knowledge and understanding needed to treat chronic kidney disease in the community. Having read it, we hope you feel confident and ready to team up with your nephrology colleagues in supporting your CKD patients to manage their long-term condition.

Acknowledgements

The authors wish to thank the National Clinical Director for Kidney Care, Dr Donal O'Donoghue, for his helpful comments.

References

Beckett, N.S., Peters, R., Fletcher, A.E. *et al.*; HYVET Study Group (2008) Treatment of hypertension in patients 80 years of age or older. *New England Journal of Medicine*, **358**, 1887–98.

Chandna, S.M., Da Silva-Gane, M., Marshall, C. *et al.* (2011) Survival of elderly patients with stage 5 CKD: comparison of conservative management and renal replacement therapy. *Nephrology, Dialysis, Transplantation*, **26**, 1608–14.

Dasgupta, I. & Rayner, H. (2009) In good conscience: withholding dialysis from the elderly. *Seminars in Dialysis*, **22**, 476–9.

Goraya, N., Simoni, J., Jo, C. & Wesson, D.E. (2012) Dietary acid reduction with fruits and vegetables or bicarbonate attenuates kidney injury in patients with a moderately reduced glomerular filtration rate due to hypertensive nephropathy. *Kidney International*, **81**, 86–93.

Hermida, R.C., Ayala, D.E., Mojón, A. & Fernández, J.R. (2011) Bedtime dosing of antihypertensive medications reduces cardiovascular risk in CKD. *Journal of the American Society of Nephrology*, **22**, 2313–21.

Rayner, H.C., Hollingworth, L., Higgins, R. & Dodds, S. (2011) Systematic kidney disease management in a population with diabetes mellitus: turning the tide of kidney failure. *BMJ Quality and Safety*, **20**, 903–10.

Stoves, J., Connolly, J., Cheung, C.K. *et al.* (2010) Electronic consultation as an alternative to hospital referral for patients with chronic kidney disease: a novel application for networked electronic health records to improve the accessibility and efficiency of healthcare. *Quality and Safety in Health Care*, **19**(5), e54. doi:10.1136/qshc.2009.038984.

UK Renal Registry (2010) 13th Annual Report 2010. http://www.renalreg.com/Reports/2010.html (accessed September 2012).

Vegter, S., Perna, A., Postma, M.J. *et al.* (2012) Sodium intake, ACE inhibition, and progression to ESRD. *Journal of the American Society of Nephrology*, **23**, 165–73.

Resources

Renal PatientView. www.renalpatientview.org (accessed September 2012).

Rare Disease UK. www.raredisease.org.uk (accessed September 2012).

AUDIT-C. www.alcohollearningcentre.org.uk/_library/AUDIT-C.doc (accessed September 2012).

Patient.co.uk. Chronic kidney disease. www.patient.co.uk/health/Chronic-Kidney-Disease.htm (accessed September 2012).

NHS Patient Decision Aids (PDAs). www.nhsdirect.nhs.uk/DecisionAids.aspx (accessed September 2012).

Chapter 4

General Considerations Related to Treatment Modalities

Aisha I. Geeson[1], Charles R. V. Tomson[1] and Lesley Lappin[2]

[1] Southmead Hospital, Bristol, UK
[2] Salford Royal NHS Foundation Trust, Salford, UK

Introduction

In the United Kingdom, 109 new patients per million population (pmp) were started on renal replacement therapy (RRT) in 2009. Ninety days after starting RRT, 47.4% of these patients were on hospital haemodialysis (HD), 25.8% were on satellite HD, 0.7% were on home HD, 18.9% were on peritoneal dialysis (PD) and 7.2% had a functioning transplant. The median age for starting RRT was 64.8 years, and 61.7% of new patients started on RRT were male. For many years, the 'take-on' rate of new patients has increased – largely because improved funding allowed patients to be offered treatment who would previously not have been offered treatment, and partly because of an ageing population and an increased prevalence of diabetes. However, for the last few years, take-on rate appears to have stabilised, and at a rate well below that of some other developed nations, such as the USA. This is likely to be due mostly to arresting the progression of CKD in primary care in the UK, but may also be due to the increasing use of maximal conservative care.

The survival of patients with chronic kidney disease (CKD) stage 3–5 is improving over time, presumably due to improvements in care. Patients aged 18–64 who started on RRT in 2004 had a five-year survival of 67.9%, compared to 60.7% for the cohort starting in 1997; and patients aged over 65 starting RRT in 2004 had a five-year survival of 26.9%, compared to 16.5% for the cohort starting in 1997. However, survival still compares poorly to that for

Kidney Disease Management: A Practical Approach for the Non-Specialist Healthcare Practitioner, First Edition. Edited by Rachel Lewis and Helen Noble.
© 2013 John Wiley & Sons, Ltd. Published 2013 by John Wiley & Sons, Ltd.

common malignant diseases: overall five-year survival for breast cancer is 83.3%, for prostate cancer 79.7%, and for colon cancer 50–52.9%.

Referral

The UK National Institute for Health and Clinical Excellence (NICE) guidelines recommend that all patients with CKD stages 4 and 5, and patients with CKD and rapidly deteriorating renal function, should be referred to, or discussed with, a nephrologist. Rapidly deteriorating renal function is defined as a fall in estimated glomerular filtration rate (eGFR) of more than $5\,mL/min/1.73\,m^2$ in 12 months or a drop in eGFR of more than $10\,mL/min/1.73\,m^2$ over five years. Additional referral criteria, designed to pick up patients likely to benefit from specialist management, include heavy proteinuria, proteinuria with haematuria, and resistant hypertension.

Late referral, usually defined as referral to a nephrologist less than 90 days before the start of RRT, is associated with higher risks of hospitalisation, complications and mortality (Chan *et al.* 2007). Late referral also prevents patients benefiting from interventions that can delay progression of their renal impairment and from pre-emptive transplantation. Late-referred patients are less likely to undergo PD, and are more likely to start HD without a functioning arteriovenous fistula. Late referrals are more common in the elderly, and may represent up to 60% of elderly patients presenting with stage 5 CKD. Reassuringly, there has been a steady fall in the number of late referrals, from 27% in 2004 to 19% in 2009, possibly due to improved recognition of high-risk patients in primary care as a result of the Quality and Outcomes Framework (QOF) and the availability of referral guidelines.

As recognition of progressive CKD improves, an increasing proportion of so-called late referrals are in fact unavoidable late presentations of kidney disease that could not reasonably have been anticipated or diagnosed earlier, for instance kidney disease caused by previously undiagnosed myeloma or systemic vasculitis. Such patients form an irreducible minimum of patients who will present as uraemic emergencies.

Variation and inequity in the use of different RRT modalities

The proportion of patients on home HD and on PD varies widely from centre to centre in the UK, and this variation cannot be explained by differences in age or comorbidity. Whether the variation is caused by supply-led demand (the economic incentive to fill HD spaces once a new satellite unit has been opened, for instance), by inadequate clinical expertise in home-based therapies, or by a genuine clinical belief (in the absence of evidence) that PD is associated with inferior clinical outcomes, is uncertain. Some variation in uptake of home-based therapies is attributable to variations in housing stock; it is much easier to establish patients on home treatment if they own their own home than if they live in multi-occupancy tenancies, for instance. Some centres have found ways to pay for carers to offer 'assisted PD', in which a carer is paid to help older, frail patients with PD at home. The numbers are currently small, but new financial arrangements may result in expansion of this modality in England.

Recent research from the UK Renal Registry has shown that social deprivation is associated with a lower chance of being put on the transplant waiting list. Once social deprivation had been taken into account, there was no association between ethnic origin and transplant listing. There is also marked centre-to-centre variation in the chances of new patients with stage 3–5 CKD being added to the transplant waiting list. The proportion of new patients under 65 years of age who are on the transplant list within two years of the start of RRT varies from less than 20% to greater than 80%. Patients looked after in non-transplanting renal centres are less likely to be placed on the transplant waiting list than those managed in transplanting renal centres. The reasons for these variations are the subject of ongoing research.

Once patients are on the transplant waiting list, the chance of receiving a transplant depends on how active the local centre is in facilitating living donor transplantation, and, at present, on the number of organs retrieved from donors after cardiac death. For the majority of patients for whom no living donor can be found, there is a national organ allocation scheme for kidneys from donors after brainstem death, described in detail below. This is designed to maximise the overall benefit from transplantation.

Empowering patients to make an informed choice: shared decision making

'Shared decision making' describes a process in which a patient chooses between different treatment options, based on a full understanding of the advantages and disadvantages of the options and on his or her own preferences and attitudes. Patients who feel that they have been part of the decision about a particular treatment are more likely to adhere to that treatment in the long term. Facilitating this type of decision making involves multidisciplinary education and the use of patient decision aids for each 'preference-sensitive decision'. Although some patients appear to prefer the team looking after them to make decisions for them, it remains important to establish the preferences of the patient when making preference-sensitive decisions, rather than imposing the preferences of the medical team (Ubel *et al*. 2011). Decision aids to support patients choosing whether or not to undergo dialysis, or choosing dialysis modality, are under development in the UK.

There is wide variation among UK centres in the quality of written information, the availability of dedicated education nurses, and the provision of structured education programmes for patients deciding on RRT modality. This variation persists despite good evidence that patients who undergo a structured education programme are more likely to choose a self-care modality (especially PD), and have better compliance and improved survival (Wingard *et al*. 2007).

Choice of RRT modality

Decisions and preparation for RRT take a long time. CKD is often an incidental finding, and remains asymptomatic until a late stage, so patients with CKD often have difficulty in accepting that they have a potentially fatal disease for which advance planning is beneficial. Delayed decisions regarding treatment modalities can result in the patient requiring emergency dialysis (due to hyperkalaemia, pulmonary oedema or pericarditis), by which time it is often too late for any real choice. These patients are likely to start HD with a temporary central venous catheter, the use of which is associated with an increased risk of infection, thrombosis, and poor flow resulting in inadequate dialysis dose. Emergency insertion of a Tenckhoff catheter for PD can be performed in such patients, but in many centres this is seldom considered.

For these reasons and others, many patients on HD report feeling that they were not given a choice of treatment. The extent to which genuine choice is offered to patients at the start of RRT has not been systematically studied in the UK. In Canada, many patients with stage 3–5 CKD report having no information about their options, whereas in Australia 84% of patients reported being presented with information about their options prior to starting dialysis. Throughout their lives, many patients with stage 5 CKD will experience several different treatment options depending on changes in their personal circumstances, while waiting for transplantation, or when one type of treatment modality fails. Instead of RRT being a choice, it can be thought of as an integrated treatment pathway. In addition, the best modality will vary from one individual to another.

Factors influencing decision making

There are several factors which influence patients when deciding on which modality they would prefer (Morton *et al.* 2010). Some patients prefer to take control of their treatment and will choose a self-care therapy. Other patients feel safer when someone medically trained carries out their treatment. Patients are sometime influenced by both the negative and positive experiences of other patients. For example, patients may decide on transplantation because they have seen another patient looking well following transplantation, or they may decide against haemodialysis when they see patients with a swollen arm following an access-related complication. (Similar considerations apply to the use of 'expert patients' in education programmes: patients are often expert in their own experiences, but do not always have sufficient knowledge of other patients' experiences, and may bring their own biases to the discussion, thus offsetting some of the benefits of being able to describe the experience of RRT first-hand.) Some patients will give more weight to survival, and others to medium-term quality of life and the effects of a treatment strategy on their current lifestyle. Some elderly patients are concerned about the burden that their treatment will place on their family members. Some patients with familial disease, for instance polycystic kidney disease, will be influenced by the experiences of other family members who have undergone RRT, often decades earlier, and it is important to explore these in detail, as the results and complications of treatment may have changed considerably since.

Cognitive impairment and lack of mental capacity

The prevalence of cognitive impairment in patients with CKD stage 3-5 is 16-38%, much higher than in the general population. Cognitive impairment is likely to affect a patient's ability to make informed decisions about whether or not to start RRT, the choice of modality, and the outcome of RRT, but is under-recognised by nephrologists. HD may accelerate the progression of vascular dementia. There is a strong case for the routine use of screening tools for cognitive impairment in pre-dialysis clinics, and an urgent need for guidelines on RRT for patients who lack capacity. Nephrologists should also encourage patients with CKD who retain mental capacity to record advance directives stating their wishes should they lose capacity.

Options

The purpose of all forms of RRT is to improve symptoms, quality of life and survival amongst patients with advanced CKD, by replacing the excretory functions of the kidney. Additional treatments are required to replace the endocrine functions of the kidney (e.g. erythropoiesis-stimulating agents to correct anaemia, hydroxylated vitamin D derivatives to correct hyperparathy-roidism and osteomalacia). Adjunctive treatments are also often required – for instance, phosphate binders are prescribed to reduce phosphate absorption from food, because removal of phosphate by most forms of dialysis is inade-quate. Antihypertensive drug treatments are often required, because RRT does not fully correct all of the factors that contribute to hypertension in CKD.

The decisions facing patients with CKD, and the professionals responsible for their care, vary over time, and include:

- whether or not to undergo RRT
- timing of the start of RRT
- whether or not to have a kidney transplant
- whether to have treatment at home, in a satellite unit or in a hospital setting
- whether to have PD or HD
- whether to withdraw from RRT

Making an informed decision requires a full understanding of the various options and their interactions with the patient's preferences, lifestyle and comorbidities – which may themselves change over time.

Timing of start

Internationally, there has been a trend towards initiating dialysis with a higher eGFR, driven partly by the recognition that clearance of small molecules is poorer in patients with advanced CKD than it is in those receiving doses of dialysis shown to confer optimal survival. In the UK, the mean eGFR at initiation of dialysis in 1999 was 6.9 mL/min/1.73 m^2 for both HD and PD, compared with more recent figures of 8.5 and 9.2 for HD and PD respectively. The Renal Association guidelines recommend that renal replacement therapy should commence when a patient has an eGFR <15 mL/min/1.73 m^2 *and* has symptoms or signs of uraemia, fluid overload or malnutrition in spite of medical therapy; or before eGFR has fallen below 6 mL/min/1.73 m^2 in an asymptomatic patient.

Early observational studies showed that earlier initiation was associated with improved survival. However, these studies failed to distinguish adequately between late presentation and late start. Later observational and registry studies have shown that there is no mortality benefit from initiating dialysis early, and many recent studies have shown higher mortality in patients starting RRT with more residual renal function than in those starting with more advanced disease. While these findings are mostly explained by the fact that patients with comorbidity often start with higher residual function than those without, it is impossible to exclude the possibility that dialysis itself might cause harm – for instance as a result of infection associated with peritoneal or vascular access, the effects of fistula formation on cardiovascular function, or the haemodynamic instability caused by dialysis treatment.

A recent randomised controlled trial which compared early start (eGFR 10-14) with late start (eGFR 5-7) showed no difference in mortality or quality of life. However, a large proportion of the patients who were assigned to the late-start group were started on dialysis earlier because of symptoms, and many in the early-start group were actually started with an eGFR <10 (Cooper *et al.* 2010).

Peritoneal dialysis

Peritoneal dialysis (PD) is the primary form of treatment used at home and for self-dialysis. The purpose of peritoneal dialysis is to remove solutes and maintain acid–base and fluid balance. Peritoneal dialysis therapy involves draining dialysis solution into the peritoneal cavity via a catheter inserted through the abdominal wall. The solution contains electrolytes and an osmotic agent – usually glucose. The peritoneal membrane is semipermeable, permitting solutes to diffuse across the membrane from the blood into the dialysis solution in the peritoneal cavity, so that draining the fluid out results in removal of these solutes, including uraemic toxins and water.

Peritoneal membrane

The peritoneal membrane is a thin, translucent, porous layer of tissue with numerous blood vessels. It consists of two layers, the parietal layer, which lines the inner surface of the abdominal wall, and the visceral layer, which covers the abdominal organs in the peritoneal cavity. The visceral peritoneum accounts for about 80% of the total peritoneal surface area. The space between the parietal and visceral peritoneum is called the peritoneal cavity. It normally contains less than 10 mL of fluid, but can accommodate several litres without patient discomfort. The osmotic gradient between plasma and dialysate also generates convective loss of water and solutes, enabling control of fluid balance.

The rapidity with which small solutes (e.g. glucose, urea) are transported across the peritoneal membrane varies markedly from patient to patient, and cannot be predicted, but has to be measured, usually six weeks after the start of PD and annually thereafter, by the peritoneal equilibration test. Fast transport results in rapid equilibration between dialysate and plasma. This results in rapid removal of urea, but also rapid loss of osmotic gradient, and eventually – if the 'dwell time' is too long – net absorption of fluid from the peritoneal cavity, resulting in low drain volumes, and thus low net removal of uraemic toxins. Slow transport allows sustained ultrafiltration, but results in slower removal of uraemic toxins. Fast transporters benefit from rapid cycles; slow transporters need fewer, longer cycles.

Additional complications are caused by the complex nature of the peritoneal membrane. Water (but not solutes) can pass through aquaporins (small pores) in the cell membrane of the peritoneal cells, whereas solutes can only pass by convection through medium and large pores between cells. Early in the cycle, particularly in slow transporters, water transport from the body into the dialysate causes hypernatraemia and a reduction of the dialysate sodium concentration, which, later in the cycle, drives convective transfer of sodium through medium pores. Using short cycles in slow transporters can thus cause hypernatraemia, resulting in thirst and compounding problems with salt and water overload (Van Biesen et al. 2010).

Peritoneal dialysis access: the Tenckhoff catheter

In 1968, Tenckhoff and Schechter revolutionised the field of PD when they introduced a permanent catheter and a method of implantation that for the first time allowed relatively long periods of usage with a significant reduction in exit-site infections. Tenckhoff recommended using a curved tunnel, downward-directed exit to reduce a potential accumulation of debris at the exit site and to reduce infection. These innovations became the basis for PD catheters still used today. Most catheters used in modern practice are silastic coiled catheters with a radiopaque marker.

Catheter insertion should be undertaken by an experienced operator, under operating-room sterile conditions. The operator can be a surgeon, specialist nurse or physician, who has specific training and expertise in peritoneal dialysis access creation. This can be done on either an inpatient or an outpatient basis. About two-thirds of catheter insertions in the UK are performed using the open surgical technique, with the majority of the others using the medical percutaneous technique, and a small number using peritoneoscopy. Catheters can be inserted under local anaesthetic, with or without sedation, or general anaesthetic. The type of anaesthetic used will depend on the method of insertion and patient comorbidities. The anaesthetic requirement for the procedure depends on the technique selected, which is influenced by the characteristics of the patient (Figueiredo *et al.* 2010).

Preoperative preparation

The Renal Association guidelines recommend that patients have their PD access surgery approximately two weeks before commencing dialysis (Woodrow & Davies 2011). Prior to surgery it is important to identify and repair any hernias. It is also important to determine where the exit site should be, this should be done with discussion with the patient so that the exit site does not sit on the belt line and the patient can see the exit site. Patients should have laxatives/bowel preparations as per local guidance. Measures should be taken to reduce the risk of infection, such as skin washing and perioperative antibiotic prophylaxis (See Chapter 7).

Once the catheter is placed, and until healing is completed, the dressing changes should be done by a dialysis nurse using an aseptic non-touch technique (Figueiredo *et al.* 2010). The area should be kept dry until it is well healed, usually for 10-14 days to permit healing and reduce the frequency of early peri-catheter leakage of dialysate. Catheters inserted percutaneously can often be used earlier than this.

On discharge home, the patient should be given laxatives with instructions to avoid constipation, and advice on recognition of potential complications.

Types of PD

Peritoneal dialysis can be performed in a number of ways, and these are described below.

Continuous ambulatory peritoneal dialysis (CAPD)

This is the most common form of PD. The process of draining and filling is called an exchange, and it takes about 30-40 minutes to complete. The period the dialysis solution is in the abdomen is called the dwell time. A typical schedule consists of approximately four two-litre dialysis exchanges a day, each with a dwell time of 4-6 hours. The last exchange of the day is usually left in overnight and exchanged the following morning. It is a simple procedure that most patients are able to perform, and there are assisted devices available for patients with visual or dexterity problems. No machines are necessary, and this procedure can be performed in many locations outside of the home, making travelling and holidays easy to organise. It is less suitable for fast transporters without residual renal function.

Automated peritoneal dialysis (APD)

APD uses an automated cycler machine to perform exchanges during the night while the patient is asleep. In the morning one exchange begins, with a dwell time that lasts the entire day. It is also sometimes called continuous cycler-assisted peritoneal dialysis (CCPD). Initially, when there is still residual renal function, it may use relatively small volumes of dialysis fluid, but as this declines, larger fill volumes and longer overnight dwells are needed. It may be particularly suitable for the young and people in full-time education or employment. The machines are portable, and, with planning, travelling and holidays are possible. APD is particularly useful for maintaining adequate control of fluid balance in fast transporters without residual renal function.

Assisted automated peritoneal dialysis (aAPD)

Assisted APD has been established in other countries for some time, but within the UK it is a relatively new concept. A healthcare assistant who has received specific basic training will visit the patient daily to prepare the APD machine. Dialysis is initiated and discontinued by the patient or family member/carer. This service allows more elderly, frail patients to continue on PD in their home environment, instead of transferring to in-centre HD.

Peritoneal dialysis solutions

Peritoneal dialysis solutions are made up of electrolytes (sodium, calcium), buffers to correct acidosis, and osmotic agents (glucose or icodextrin) to drive fluid removal. At present, commercially available solutions do not offer a choice of sodium concentration, although research into the potential advantages of low-sodium dialysate on fluid balance and blood pressure is being undertaken. Calcium content can be 1.25 or 1.75 mmol/L; the choice depends on local policy for bone mineral disease management.

Most commercially available peritoneal dialysis solutions contain lactate as the buffer. It is absorbed into the systemic circulation and is converted by the liver to bicarbonate. Bicarbonate cannot routinely be used in dialysis solutions because it crystallises with calcium and magnesium during storage. Solutions with dual chambers have been designed to get round this problem. The bicarbonate is mixed with the dialysate just before the fluid is used.

Glucose is the main osmotic agent used in peritoneal dialysis solution. Three strengths of glucose solution (low, medium and high) are available. Fluid removal goes up with the strength of bag used.

Icodextrin is a larger glucose polymer and is not associated with systemic absorption. Its use results in slow ultrafiltration over a long dwell time. Its use is favoured in fast transporters who have inadequate ultrafiltration.

Fluid balance, residual renal function, ultrafiltration failure

The importance of fluid management for patient outcome has been repeatedly demonstrated. Fluid overload is associated with adverse cardiovascular outcomes including hypertension and left ventricular hypertrophy. If too much fluid is removed, causing hypovolaemia, this can adversely affect residual renal function. Fluid balance assessment is challenging and comprises assessment of jugular venous pressure, chest auscultation, checking for oedema, weight change and blood pressure. High blood pressure may be the only sign of fluid overload in some patients. Fluid balance is maintained by clear instructions to patients on dietary sodium and water intake, the use of diuretics, and the dialysis prescription.

Residual renal function helps to maintain fluid balance; patients with a lower urine output require stricter restriction of oral fluid intake. The largest change in urine output is usually observed in the first month of therapy as PD corrects the polyuria of chronic kidney disease by reducing the osmotic load and extracellular volume expansion. Subsequent changes in urine output are usually slowly progressive except during episodes of acute illness such as peritonitis, when nephrotoxic agents are used, or in situations that cause fluctuations in blood pressure.

Patients are encouraged to weigh themselves daily to help with fluid assessment, and should be educated about the symptoms of hypovolaemia and fluid overload. It is important to give clear instructions to patients about fluid intake, and this will change over time as residual renal function tails off. Fluid overload can be caused by non-concordance with dietary sodium and water recommendations or diuretics, by incorrect dialysis prescription or by ultrafiltration failure. Extra fluid can be removed by adjusting the dialysis prescription – by changing the solutions, switching PD modality or altering the number of exchanges. Dialysis solutions with higher glucose concentration or icodextrin can remove extra fluid. Although high-strength bags are useful for rapid correction of fluid overload, routine use is not recommended, as higher-strength bags are associated with more metabolic complications from glucose absorption (e.g. hyperglycaemia, hyperinsulinaemia, hyperlipidaemia and weight gain) and greater peritoneal membrane injury.

Training and education for PD patients

Education is key to the success of home dialysis therapy (Woodrow & Davies 2011). Patients are taught about all aspects of their dialysis by specialist nurses, either in-centre or in their home environment. Healthcare providers have a responsibility to provide appropriate and individualised education in all aspects of PD to ensure that the patient is fully engaged with his or her care. This helps to avoid complications. Patient education must include instruction on aseptic measures to prevent infection, the timing and number of exchanges to be performed, appropriate dwell times, use of the cycler if automated dialysis is chosen, obtaining the proper dialysate solutions, storage of solutions and equipment and fluid balance. Troubleshooting potential problems and 'What to do if ...' advice should be incorporated into the training period.

It can take 3–5 days of training before patients are fully conversant in all aspects of their PD and feel confident to undertake the dialysis procedure themselves. In some centres, carers are taught how to perform PD as well as the patient. Education and support is provided on a continuous basis, and is reinforced after any episodes of infection or inter-current problems.

Common complications and treatments

Irrespective of where CKD patients are managed and by whom, it is recommended practice to consult the renal team for clinical management advice for renal-related problems. The renal team should be informed immediately of any dialysis patient requiring urgent hospital admission.

Infectious complications of PD

Peritonitis

The most common serious complication of PD is peritonitis, an infection of the peritoneum. This significantly contributes to technique failure and hospitalisation. Peritonitis is usually caused by bacteria getting into the peritoneum via the dialysis catheter, usually due to touch contamination during the dialysis exchange. Skin bacteria or fungi can cause the infection. Peritonitis in patients receiving PD usually occurs within 48 hours of contamination. Occasionally, peritonitis can be caused by bowel disease (e.g. diverticulitis), and this should be suspected if multiple bowel organisms are identified on culture.

Patients with peritonitis usually present with cloudy dialysate effluent, first noticed when the fluid has been drained out of the peritoneal cavity during the exchange procedure. Abdominal pain may or may not be present during early presentation. Peritonitis should always be included in the differential diagnosis of the PD patient with abdominal pain, even if the dialysate effluent is clear. An elevated dialysate count of white blood cells of more than $100/mm^3$, of which at least 50% are polymorphonuclear neutrophils, is supportive of the diagnosis of bacterial peritonitis, and calls for immediate initiation of antimicrobial therapy (Li *et al.* 2010). Effective treatment for PD-associated peritonitis is necessary to reduce morbidity and possibly mortality associated with the acute episode and to reduce relapse rates. Severe and prolonged peritonitis can lead to peritoneal membrane failure.

A wide variety of antimicrobial agents have been used successfully for the treatment of peritonitis, including the glycopeptides, penicillins, cephalosporins, aminoglycosides and fluoroquinolones. Intraperitoneal (IP) administration is the most common method used because, given adequate dwell times, it achieves high local drug concentrations and permits self-treatment by the patient; however, oral and intravenous (IV) administration have also been used. Ideally, antibiotic treatment of PD peritonitis would be guided by Gram stain and/or dialysate culture results. This is impractical because it requires a delay in commencement of treatment. Therefore, it is necessary for each PD unit to have a standard empirical drug regimen with which to start treatment. This regimen can then be adjusted at a later stage if indicated by culture results.

Generally, if a patient is demonstrating signs of an 'acute' abdomen, the possibility of bowel perforation or abdominal obstruction cannot be ruled out. Further investigations, along with a surgical opinion, should be sought, and the patient requires urgent admission.

PD services are usually based on specialist nurse interventions, and with a well-defined protocol as a framework for management most episodes of peritonitis can be dealt with on an outpatient basis. The patient's dialysis technique should be reassessed by the specialist nurse, and further education and training can be carried out as necessary.

Indications for catheter removal in patients with PD peritonitis include catheter or tunnel infection, fungal, tuberculous, persistent or relapsing peritonitis, bowel perforations, cuff erosion and protrusion, and post-transplant peritonitis.

Exit-site infections

An exit-site infection is defined by the presence of purulent drainage, with or without erythema of the skin, at the catheter–epidermal interface. Pericatheter erythema without purulent drainage is sometimes an early indication of infection but can also be a simple skin reaction, particularly in a recently placed catheter or after trauma to the catheter. Clinical judgement is required to decide whether to initiate therapy or monitor closely (Li *et al.* 2010). Community staff should consult local specialist services, as most centres have their own protocol for the management of PD access-related infections.

Routine screening

Routine screening for nasal, groin, axillary and exit site of staphyloccocal carriage is performed, and if positive treatment with mupirocin and octenisan is performed as per local protocols. Some units are now screening for and treating exit-site *Pseudomonas* colonisation.

Non-infectious complications of PD

Hypoalbuminaemia

Albumin loss is seen due to high protein losses in the dialysate, especially during episodes of peritonitis. These losses can be as high as 10–20 g a day, and patients may require protein supplementation either orally or intravenously.

Electrolyte and acid–base disturbances

Hypernatraemia can occur as a result of sodium sieving, as described above. Hyponatraemia can occur as a result of excessive thirst (possibly caused by over-aggressive fluid removal) or total body potassium depletion. Lactic acidosis is rare except in patients with terminal liver failure, and can be avoided by the use of bicarbonate-containing peritoneal dialysis fluid. Occasionally, severe lactic acidosis can be due to ongoing bowel ischemia, and this should be excluded under relevant clinical conditions.

Catheter-related complications: placement, hernia, malfunction

Patients can present with problems with draining fluid in or out. Problems with draining can be related to catheter malposition, constipation or blocked catheter from fibrin or omental wrapping. An abdominal x-ray is useful to confirm the position of the tube and would also show whether the patient is constipated. Simple laxatives can help, or, if tube position is a problem, then repositioning or replacement can be carried. If catheter occlusion is suspected, then injecting fibrin or heparin through the catheter may be useful.

Fluid leaks

Fluid leaks can present in a number of ways depending on where the leak is. Peri-catheter leaks will result in wet dressings, abdominal wall oedema or genital oedema. Genital oedema can also be caused by fluid leaking into an inguinal hernia.

Investigation of suspected leaks will vary between units depending on local expertise but may include a CT or x-ray with intraperitoneal contrast, or an MRI. If a leak is suspected or confirmed, the peritoneum should be rested to allow the membrane to heal, and PD should be restarted with low volumes. Persistent leaks may require a surgical repair or the catheter to be changed.

Encapsulating peritoneal sclerosis

Encapsulating peritoneal sclerosis (EPS) is a rare and serious complication of PD. The peritoneal membrane becomes fibrotic and the intestines become embedded in this fibrous tissue. Patients can present with malnutrition, bowel obstruction, abdominal pain and problems with PD. A CT scan should be performed to help with diagnosis. If EPS is confirmed then PD should be stopped. Malnutrition may have to be managed with total parenteral nutrition (TPN). Surgery may be indicated in some cases, and should only be performed in designated specialist centres.

Haemodialysis, haemofiltration and haemodiafiltration

The purpose of dialysis is to remove waste products from the body, to correct electrolyte and acid base abnormalities, and to maintain fluid balance. The removal of solute and fluid occurs by diffusion and convection.

Haemodialysis

Haemodialysis (HD) involves pumping blood through an array of hollow fibres made of a semipermeable material, while pumping dialysate (a solution of highly purified water, sodium, chloride, magnesium, dextrose and bicarbonate or acetate) in the opposite direction around the outside of the fibres (counter-current flow). This allows molecules and electrolytes to diffuse across from the blood into the dialysate and vice versa, with the countercurrent flow maximising the concentration gradients at all points along the fibre. Net fluid removal is achieved by altering the hydrostatic pressures in the blood and dialysate compartments, causing convective flow of plasma water, together with any molecules big enough to cross the membrane. The dialysis machine controls the chemical composition of the dialysate (by proportionating highly purified water with concentrates of the chemicals required), the blood and dialysate pressure, and the flow rates.

Haemofiltration

Haemofiltration is predominantly used in the critical care setting. Convection rather than diffusion is used to remove solutes and fluid. The fluid is then replaced by large volumes of a substitution fluid. Typically, 1–2 litres is exchanged each hour.

Haemodiafiltration

Haemodiafiltration is a combination of haemodialysis and haemofiltration. Typically, 'online' preparation of the substitution fluid is used, analogous to the way in which dialysate is used, in preference to the use of large volumes of fluid in bags; however, because the substitution fluid is to be infused directly into the patient, purity and freedom from bacteriological contamination is even more important, requiring additional water purification steps. Some units favour the use of haemodiafiltration over haemodialysis because it may reduce the frequency and severity of intra-dialytic and post-dialytic adverse symptoms and may be more effective than HD in the removal of middle molecules and phosphate. A Cochrane review has concluded that there is no evidence to support this, but further studies are needed (Rabindranath *et al.* 2006).

Membrane

The membrane in the dialyser can be cellulose, modified cellulose or synthetic. Modified cellulose and synthetic membrane are more biocompatible than cellulose membranes and can both be high flux. This means that they are associated with less inflammation and greater clearance of larger solutes such a beta-2 microglobulin.

High flux versus low flux

High-flux dialysis is generally considered for use in patients who are unlikely to be transplanted, to delay the complications associated with long-term dialysis, such as cardiovascular disease and dialysis-related amyloidosis (Tattersall *et al.* 2009) . The HEMO study showed high-flux dialysis to be associated with increased clearance of middle molecules, but did not show any survival benefit (Eknoyan *et al.* 2002). However, secondary analysis has shown a survival advantage with high-flux dialysis in patients who have been on dialysis for >3.7 years. The MPO study showed a possible advantage of high flux for patients with diabetes and those with hypoalbuminaemia (Locatelli *et al.* 2009).

Vascular access

There are three main types of vascular access: central venous catheter (tunnelled or non-tunnelled), arteriovenous fistula or graft. A native arteriovenous fistula is the preferred method of dialysis access because fistulae are associated with the highest blood flow rates and consequently better solute clearance, the lowest rates of infection and thrombosis, and the greatest longevity. The drawback of arteriovenous fistulae is that they are associated with higher rates of primary failure and take longer to mature. They are usually ready to use after six weeks, compared with two weeks for PTFE grafts.

Hospital, satellite or home haemodialysis?

Haemodialysis can be performed in hospital, in a satellite unit or at home. Patients who are dialysed in hospital or a satellite unit usually have three sessions per week, each lasting 4–5 hours. Home haemodialysis is more flexible. Some patients opt for thrice-weekly dialysis, as in hospital or satellite dialysis. However, if funding permits, many patients opt for daily short dialysis, usually 1.5–2 hours daily, or for nocturnal dialysis, usually 7–8 hours each night with a slow pump speed. Nocturnal HD is associated with increased solute clearance, better phosphate control, better blood pressure control, with many patients coming off all antihypertensives, and regression of left ventricular hypertrophy. However, further research is needed to assess the impact of nocturnal dialysis on survival.

Self-care dialysis within a satellite unit is an emerging option, in which patients use a satellite dialysis unit to dialyse in but take full responsibility for their own treatment, including preparation of the machine, needling the fistula, management of the dialysis session, and stripping the machine at completion. Provision of dedicated facilities for self-care dialysis can also allow patients to arrange their own dialysis schedules, with some of the flexibility associated with home treatment.

'Dose' of haemodialysis

Haemodialysis removes hundreds of substances that accumulate in stage 5 CKD, many of which do not even have names. The efficiency with which these substances are removed varies according to the type of dialysis membrane used, the relative contribution of convection and diffusion, the flow rates of blood and dialysate, and the efficiency with which blood returning from the dialyser mixes with the rest of the patient's bloodstream. In routine clinical practice, the dose of haemodialysis is prescribed to achieve adequate clearance of urea – an easily measured small molecule that reaches high concentrations in kidney failure. The percentage reduction in blood urea concentration during a dialysis session (the urea reduction ratio, URR) is the simplest index of urea removal, but does not take account of urea removed by convection. The Kt/V_{urea} expresses the ratio *volume of blood cleared of urea : urea distribution volume* and can be accurately measured only by iterative computerised modelling with numerous inputs including the *in vitro* dialyser urea clearance and measurements of the inter-dialytic urea generation rate, but can be estimated by simplified formulae that require, for example, pre- and post-dialysis urea concentration, time on dialysis and ultrafiltration volume. All measurements that involve the post-dialysis urea concentration are susceptible to errors caused by rapid rebound in urea concentration as dialysed blood equilibrates fully within the body. Kt/V formulae therefore refer either to 'single pool' or 'equilibrated' Kt/V (SpKt/V, eKt/V). Current clinical practice guidelines state that patients on thrice-weekly haemodialysis should have dialysis dose measured monthly, and should achieve an eKt/V of 1.2, or a URR of >65% (Mactier *et al.* 2011).

Transplantation

Fitness for transplantation

The purpose of transplantation is to improve survival and quality of life. Therefore, it is important to assess whether the potential recipient is fit for major surgery and chronic immunosuppression. Pre-transplant workup involves an assessment of the patient's cardiovascular risk (the extent of investigation depends upon the individual's cardiovascular risk factors, including age, smoking, obesity and diabetes); peripheral vascular disease risk; lung and liver disease; and chronic infections. Many centres refuse transplantation to patients with obesity, because of the higher risk of surgical complications.

Patients with a history of malignant disease require careful assessment of whether the risk of recurrence would be increased by anti-rejection treatment. Patients who have had a non-melanoma skin cancer or in situ carcinoma of the cervix or bladder are at low risk of recurrence and can therefore be placed on the waiting list once treatment is complete. For all other malignancies, patients should have been in remission for five years. Discussion with an oncologist is advised. Age alone does not preclude transplantation, and each case is assessed individually, bearing in mind that the aim of transplantation is to improve survival and quality of life.

Once patients are considered to be fit for transplant, they should ideally be placed on the transplant list six months prior to requiring dialysis (Dudley and Harden 2011). Their ongoing fitness should be reassessed at regular intervals.

Transplant type and timing

Renal transplants can come from living, heart-beating (donor after brainstem death, DBD) or non-heart-beating (donor after cardiac death, DCD) donors. In the UK in 2010/11, a total of 2388 adult transplants were carried out; 40% were from living donors, 38% from heart-beating donors and 22% from non-heart-beating donors (NHS Blood and Transplant statistics). Transplantation can be carried out before the patient is on dialysis (pre-emptively) or after. To increase the chance of being offered a kidney, patients can choose to be considered for kidneys from 'extended criteria donors' which include kidneys from donors over the age of 60 or over the age of 50 with two of the following features: a history of hypertension, death by cerebrovascular accident, terminal creatinine >133 mmol/L.

ABO and HLA matching

The potential recipient's blood group is routinely checked during pre-transplant assessment, because ABO incompatibility can result in hyperacute rejection and graft loss.

Human leucocyte antigen (HLA) typing at three loci of the major histocompatibility complex (HLA-A/B/DR) is also routinely checked. The donor and recipient can be completely matched at the three loci (mismatch 000) or can have varying degrees of mismatch – for example, two mismatches at HLA-A, one mismatch at HLA-B and no mismatches at HLA-DR (mismatch 2,1,0). When patients are placed on the transplant waiting list a minimum mismatch score is specified. The degree of mismatches and the loci have varying degrees of influence on outcome, with mismatches at HLA-DR having the worst outcome, followed by HLA-B and HLA-A.

In addition, some patients develop antibodies to HLA antigens from blood transfusions, during pregnancy or from previous transplantation. The presence of an antibody to an HLA antigen present on a transplanted kidney predicts immediate, 'hyperacute' rejection. Potential recipients are therefore routinely tested for the presence of antibodies to HLA antigens and 'unacceptable antigens' are identified. These are then compared with a panel of around 10 000 donor HLA types on a national database. Patients who have antibodies against ≥85% of these HLA antigens are considered 'highly sensitised', which means that they are less likely to get a kidney. These patients are therefore given priority in the national organ allocation scheme. Prior to transplantation, a final cross-match is checked to make sure that there are no further unidentified or unacceptable antigens.

Allocation scheme

The kidneys of a DCD donor are allocated locally to minimise cold ischaemic time. However, kidneys from DBD donors are allocated nationally. There is disparity in waiting time for patients with different blood groups. In the UK, between 2004 and 2008, the mean waiting time for kidneys from blood group A was 925 days, blood group B was 1329 days, blood group AB was 655 days and O was 1381 days (UK transplant statistics). Consequently, kidneys from donors with blood group O are only allocated to recipients with blood group O, and donors with blood group B are only allocated to recipients with blood group B. The exception to this is paediatric patients and those with a complete match (mismatch 000), as discussed in more detail below.

The national allocation scheme operated by NHS Blood and Transplant works through five tiers when allocating a kidney:

Tier 1 - 000 mismatched paediatric patients: highly sensitised or HLA-DR homozygous

Tier 2 - 000 mismatched paediatric patients: others

Tier 3 - 000 mismatched adult patients: highly sensitised or HLA-DR homozygous

Tier 4 - 000 mismatched adult patients: others and favourably matched paediatric patients (100, 010, 110 mismatches)

Tier 5 - All other eligible patients

Paediatric patients in the top two tiers are prioritised according to waiting time. In the remaining tiers, potential recipients are allocated a score based on waiting time, HLA match and age combined, donor–recipient age difference, location of patient relative to donor, HLA-DR homozygosity, HLA-B homozygosity and blood group match. Rare HLA types in the recipient, commonly found in people of ethnic minority origin, are 'defaulted' to more common types to reduce the disadvantage experienced by this group of patients.

Immunosuppression and prophylaxis

In order to prevent rejection, patients are started on immunosuppressants. Patients receiving a kidney from a live donor are started on immunosuppression a few days before the transplant. Those receiving from a deceased donor will commence immunosuppression on arrival to hospital. The regime will vary depending on local protocols. In addition, recipients are given prophylaxis against opportunistic infections such as cytomegalovirus, *Pneumocystis jirovecii* pneumonia and tuberculosis. Following transplantation, patients are closely monitored for signs of rejection and toxicity from immunosuppression (Sayegh & Carpenter 2004).

Availability and waiting time

The demand for kidneys consistently exceeds the number of available deceased-donor organs. The number of patents on the UK transplant waiting list on 1 April 2009 was 9111. A further 3256 patients were added over the next 12 months, making a total of 12 367 patients. Of these, 2337 were transplanted, 327 died, and 489 were removed from the list, resulting in 9214 patients remaining active on the waiting list on 31 March 2010. This resulted in a net increase of 103 patients on the waiting list over the 12-month period.

Overall, the number of deceased-donor organs is rising. The number of DBD donors has steadily fallen over the last 10–15 years, but has now stabilised. This is partially related to a fall in head trauma secondary to road traffic accidents. In contrast, DCD donor numbers have been rising over the last 10 years. Up to 40% of potential deceased donors do not become donors because of lack of consent from relatives. The number of living kidney donors has also increased over the last 10 years, from 372 in 2000/01 to 1037 in 2009/10. In the UK the most realistic options to expand organ donation are to alter public attitudes to donation after death, particularly amongst minority populations, and to increase the number of living-donor kidney transplantations.

To expand the supply of live kidney donors, paired exchange programmes have been established so that a patient with a potential donor who is an unsuitable match can exchange kidneys with another pair in a similar position so that all recipients can receive a suitable match. In addition, some centres are now carrying out live-donor transplants across HLA and blood group barriers, using plasmapheresis to remove antibodies and a combination of agents directed against B and T lymphocytes to prevent their re-synthesis.

Conservative care

Some patients may choose not to undergo RRT, particularly (but not exclusively) in the presence of significant comorbidity. It is important to discuss with these patients and their families what their wishes are with regards to where they would like to die and to try and resolve any outstanding issues. It is also important to involve the general practitioner and palliative care so that appropriate support can be given to the patient and family and the patient receives adequate symptom control (see Chapter 10).

Survival

Since the main purpose of RRT is to prolong life amongst patients who would otherwise die from kidney failure, survival is an important outcome measure. However, comparison of survival on different types of RRT is extremely difficult, because other characteristics that determine survival – age, fitness, comorbidity – also have a major influence on which modalities a given patient might be offered, and which is then chosen. Even comparisons of survival between RRT and conservative management are complex, because most patients start RRT with some residual renal function, and are therefore not at imminent risk of death from kidney impairment. Very few randomised controlled trials have compared survival on different forms of treatment, and such trials are very difficult to design, because many patients are unwilling to be randomly allocated to treatments with such different impacts on lifestyle.

Transplant versus HD/PD

Patients who are placed on the transplant waiting list are usually younger and have fewer comorbidities than those who are not listed. The patients who are subsequently transplanted have a survival advantage over those who remain on the transplant waiting list. This is true regardless of gender, ethnicity or cause of kidney disease. Transplantation before reaching stage 5 CKD is associated with improved transplant survival compared to transplantation after 3–4 years of dialysis. The transplanted kidney and patient survival is better for a live kidney transplant compared to transplantation with a deceased-donor organ. The UK 10-year graft survival for a live kidney donation (LKD) is 79%, compared with 70% for DCD and 69% for DBD. The 10-year patient survival is 90% for LKD, 74% for DBD and 66% for DCD.

There is conflicting evidence, nearly certainly due to selection bias, on the survival of elderly patients following transplantation. In the USA the survival advantage conferred by transplantation was also present in patients aged 60–74 years. However, a UK study has shown that in patients over the age of 65 with multiple comorbidities transplantation of any kind carries more risk than benefit.

HD versus PD

In general, patients starting PD are younger, less likely to have comorbidity, and usually start RRT with a higher level of residual renal function. Most late-referred patients are started on HD, often with temporary vascular access. For these reasons and others, comparisons of outcome using observational datasets are difficult to interpret (Noordzij & Jager 2012). After adjusting for these differences, many studies suggest a modest survival advantage for PD compared to HD for at least the first year of treatment, although PD may be associated with poorer survival in patients with coronary artery disease, heart failure and diabetes.

CAPD versus APD

Overall there is no difference in survival or technique failure between patients treated with CAPD and APD. However, fast transporters have a survival advantage on APD treatment compared with CAPD, whereas slow transporters may do better on CAPD.

Home HD versus in-centre HD

Observational studies have shown that home HD is associated with better survival then in-centre HD. The studies have corrected for comorbidity in their analysis, but selection bias cannot be excluded, as the type of patient who opts for home HD is different to the patient who opts for hospital HD. In addition, quality of life is better on home HD.

Elderly patients, comorbidities and RRT

Elderly patients on dialysis survive longer than patients who are managed conservatively (Carson *et al.* 2009), but in the presence of significant comorbidity or frailty many of the additional days of life conferred by dialysis are spent in hospital. In addition, elderly dialysis patients are more likely to die in a hospital setting compared with conservatively managed patients. For all of these reasons, the decision on whether or not to undergo dialysis is particularly sensitive to patients' preferences. Some may wish to prolong survival even at the expense of a high burden of treatment and risk of hospitalisation, for instance if they are keen to stay alive to reach an anniversary, the birth of a grandchild, or other important occasion; others will opt for conservative care.

Health-related quality of life

Health-related quality of life in patients on dialysis is compromised compared with that of the general population and that of kidney transplant recipients. Patient-reported health-related quality of life is an independent predictor of survival. Patients who are transplanted have a better quality of life than those who remain on dialysis. There is conflicting evidence comparing the quality of life of patients on HD compared with PD. Home therapies are associated with a better quality of life, although patients dialysing at home tend to be younger and have fewer comorbidities. These comparisons may also be subject to selection bias, in that the psychological make-up of patients prepared to train for home dialysis may differ from that of those who prefer to cede control to others. Quality of life amongst elderly patients on PD is at least as good as in those on in-centre HD.

Psychological/emotional issues

The prevalence of depression is 27% in dialysis patients and 21% in patients with CKD. Depression is often poorly recognised because of the overlap of the psychosomatic symptoms of depression and those of uraemia, and it is consequently under-treated. Therefore it may be useful to screen for depression in both CKD and dialysis patients. Depression has been shown to adversely affect concordance and survival. Early referral, pre-dialysis education programmes, and exercise training programmes are all associated with improved mental health. Whether treatment of depression (with counselling, psychological interventions, exercise or antidepressant treatment) improves outcomes remains uncertain.

Physical issues

The physical health of dialysis patients is adversely affected by the burden of dialysis itself and by comorbidities. It has been reported that physical well-being has the greatest impact on health-related quality of life. A systematic review found that there is a great burden of symptoms in dialysis patients (Murtagh *et al*. 2007). Fatigue was found in 71%, pruritus in 55%, constipation in 53%, anorexia in 49%, pain in 47%, sleep disturbance in 44%, dyspnoea in 35%, nausea in 33% and restless legs in 30%.

Functional status

Elderly patients, both residential-home and nursing-home residents, commenced on dialysis have progressive loss of independence and functional status. In addition, few elderly diabetic patients on HD conduct any substantive portion of their lives outside their home, whereas patients who are managed with maximum conservative management maintain their functional status up until the final month of their life (Murtagh *et al*. 2011). Some nephrologists believe that instead of withholding RRT, we should be concentrating on rehabilitating these patients and optimising their nutritional status so they can maintain their functional status.

Social/occupational issues

Employment amongst patients with chronic kidney disease is nearly half of that of the age-matched general population and falls further after starting dialysis. People who receive pre-dialysis education are more likely to continue in work.

Withdrawal from RRT

From a legal point of view, patients can refuse medical treatment such as dialysis, and it is not uncommon for patients to feel that their quality of life on dialysis is so poor that they would prefer to withdraw and die. Patients may feel like this because they are not thriving on dialysis or because of a general deterioration secondary to their comorbidities. In fact withdrawal from dialysis is the third most common cause of death, accounting for 14% of deaths amongst dialysis patients in the UK in 2009. Following withdrawal, patients usually die within 7–14 days depending on residual renal function. It is important for patients to be given symptomatic relief, and that their wishes are respected to ensure that they die with dignity. Patients and their families should be involved in discussions regarding end-of-life care.

The decision to withdraw from dialysis is difficult to make. In certain cases, patients may not have the capacity to make decisions regarding their care. Some of these patients may have advance directives in which they will have documented their wishes, or they may have appointed a designated person to make decisions for them. For those who do not have the capacity to make decisions about their care and who do not have advance directives, it is important to engage in discussions with family members to try to find out what the patient would have wanted. It is important to ensure that the patient has capacity, and that inter-current depression is treated.

Increasingly, patients who are thought to be in the final year of their life are placed on a register which is shared with general practitioners and which hopefully will help to identify those who are not thriving and allow for the primary care and secondary teams to liaise in providing care (see Chapter 10).

Effective use of limited resources

The management of CKD is disproportionately costly in comparison to other medical conditions. The total cost to the UK National Health Service (NHS) of treating people who require RRT has been estimated at 1-2% of the total NHS budget, yet they comprise only 0.05% of the total population. A recent study comparing the costs of the different modalities found that the cost per year was £15570 for CAPD, £21655 for APD, £32669 for satellite haemodialysis and £35023 for hospital haemodialysis (Baboolal et al. 2008). Although CAPD is a cheaper option than other forms of dialysis, treatment decisions are generally based on a number of factors, not least the clinical effectiveness of interventions.

Transplantation costs about the same as haemodialysis in the first year. The costs include the operation, immunosuppressive drugs and regular checks. However the cost reduces considerably in subsequent years. The cost saving of kidney transplantation compared to dialysis over a period of 10 years is approximately £24100 per year for each year that the patient has a functioning transplanted kidney.

Conclusions

In conclusion, it is important for the multidisciplinary team to have regular, ongoing discussions with patients regarding their condition and available treatment options. Decision support will not only help to improve concordance and general wellbeing on dialysis but also helps patients to make informed choices that they will not later regret.

References

Baboolal, K., McEwan, P., Sondhi, S. et al. (2008) The cost of renal dialysis in a UK setting: a multicentre study. Nephrology, Dialysis, Transplantation, 23, 1982-9.

Carson, R.C., Juszczak, M., Davenport, A. & Burns, A. (2009) Is maximum conservative management an equivalent treatment option to dialysis for elderly patients with significant comorbid disease? Clinical Journal of the American Society of Nephrology, 4, 1611-19.

Chan, M.R., Dall, A.T., Fletcher, K.E., Lu, N. & Trivedi, H. (2007) Outcomes in patients with chronic kidney disease referred late to nephrologists: a meta-analysis. American Journal of Medicine, 120, 1063-70.

Cooper, B.A., Branley, P., Bulfone, L. et al. (2010) A randomized, controlled trial of early versus late initiation of dialysis. New England Journal of Medicine, 363, 609-19.

Dudley, C. & Harden, P. (2011) Renal Association clinical practice guideline on the assessment of the potential kidney transplant recipient. *Nephron Clinical Practice*, **118** (Suppl. 1), c209–24.

Eknoyan, G., Beck, G.J., Cheung, A.K. *et al.* (2002) Effect of dialysis dose and membrane flux in maintenance hemodialysis. *New England Journal of Medicine*, **347**, 2010–19.

Figueiredo, A., Goh, B.L., Jenkins, S. *et al.* (2010) Clinical practice guidelines for peritoneal access. *Peritoneal Dialysis International*, **30**, 424–9.

Li, P.K., Szeto, C.C., Piraino, B. *et al.* (2010) Peritoneal dialysis-related infections recommendations: 2010 update. *Peritoneal Dialysis International*, **30**, 393–423.

Locatelli, F., Martin-Malo, A., Hannedouche, T. *et al.*, for the Membrane Permeability Outcome (MPO) Study Group (2009) Effect of membrane permeability on survival of hemodialysis patients. *Journal of the American Society of Nephrology*, **20**, 645–54.

Mactier, R., Hoenich, N. & Breen, C. (2011) Renal Association clinical practice guideline on haemodialysis. *Nephron Clinical Practice*, **118** (Suppl. 1), c241–86.

Morton, R.L., Tong, A., Howard, K., Snelling, P. & Webster, A.C. (2010) The views of patients and carers in treatment decision making for chronic kidney disease: systematic review and thematic synthesis of qualitative studies. *BMJ*, **340**, c112.

Murtagh, F.E., Addington-Hall, J. & Higginson, I.J. (2007) The prevalence of symptoms in end-stage renal disease: a systematic review. *Advances in Chronic Kidney Disease*, **14**, 82–99.

Murtagh, F.E., Addington-Hall, J.M. & Higginson, I.J. (2011) End-stage renal disease: a new trajectory of functional decline in the last year of life. *Journal of the American Geriatrics Society*, **59**, 304–8.

Noordzij, M. & Jager, K.J. (2012) Survival comparisons between haemodialysis and peritoneal dialysis. *Nephrology, Dialysis, Transplantation* [Epub ahead of print].

Rabindranath, K.S., Strippoli, G.F., Daly, C. *et al.* (2006) Haemodiafiltration, haemofiltration and haemodialysis for end-stage kidney disease. *Cochrane Database of Systematic Reviews*, (4), CD006258.

Sayegh, M.H. & Carpenter, C.B. (2004) Transplantation 50 years later: progress, challenges, and promises. *New England Journal of Medicine*, **351**, 2761–6.

Tattersall, J., Canaud, B., Heimburger, O. *et al.* (2009) High-flux or low-flux dialysis: a position statement following publication of the Membrane Permeability Outcome study. *Nephrology, Dialysis, Transplantation*, **25**, 1230–2.

Ubel, P.A., Angott, A.M. & Zikmund-Fisher, B.J. (2011) Physicians recommend different treatments for patients than they would choose for themselves. *Archives of Internal Medicine*, **171**, 630–4.

Van Biesen, W., Heimburger, O., Krediet, R. *et al.* (2010) Evaluation of peritoneal membrane characteristics: clinical advice for prescription management by the ERBP working group. *Nephrology, Dialysis, Transplantation*, **25**, 2052–62.

Wingard, R.L., Pupim, L.B., Krishnan, M. *et al.* (2007) Early intervention improves mortality and hospitalization rates in incident hemodialysis patients: RightStart program. *Clinical Journal of the American Society of Nephrology*, **2**, 1170–5.

Woodrow, G. & Davies, S. (2011) Renal Association clinical practice guideline on peritoneal dialysis. *Nephron Clinical Practice*, **118** (Suppl. 1), c287–310.

Chapter 5

Psychosocial Aspects of Living with Chronic Kidney Disease

Emma Coyne

Nottingham University Hospitals NHS Trust, Nottingham, UK

Introduction

Living with chronic kidney disease (CKD) is a psychologically and socially challenging journey for patients, family and friends. This chapter aims to highlight some of the psychosocial issues patients may face at different stages of their renal journey, whether they are preparing for renal replacement therapy (RRT) or have chosen a conservative management pathway. It also aims to highlight the role all staff have in supporting people with CKD and when specialist psychological support may be required.

CKD and psychosocial distress

Given the impact a health problem can potentially have on a person's quality of life, it is perhaps not surprising that chronic health conditions are associated with increased levels of distress and mental health difficulties compared to the general population (NICE 2009). Prevalence rates of common mental health difficulties such as anxiety and depression in people with stage 5 CKD are high, and some estimates suggest they are higher than in other chronic conditions. Approximately 25% of people with CKD may be struggling with clinically significant symptoms of depression, and prevalence rates on commencing dialysis may be over 40% (Watnick *et al.* 2003, Ver Halen *et al.* 2012). Many people with CKD i.e. stress will be faced with more general, subclinical psychosocial difficulties at some point during their lifetime. There are a number of possible reasons for this including the impact of physical

Table 5.1 A biopsychosocial understanding of a person with CKD.

The person with chronic kidney disease			
Biological factors	Psychological factors	Social factors	Environmental factors
Chronic kidney disease	Core beliefs about self, others, world	Close family • Parents • Siblings • Partner/spouse • Children • Grandchildren	Societal expectations
Comorbid health conditions, e.g. diabetes	Personality		Culture
	Health locus of control		Age-related expectations
Genetic disorders	Self-efficacy		Cultural attitudes and awareness/ stigma towards CKD
Infection	Mood	Wider family	
Anaemia	Emotions, e.g. guilt, shame	Education	
Hormonal conditions		Work/activity	
Immune response	Illness representations	Hobbies	Housing
Organic brain issues		Financial situation	Transport
Medication (effects and side-effects)	Resilience	Social support/ friends	Healthcare system
Current treatment e.g. dialysis, transplant	Adjustment to health problems	Access to health care	
	Concordance issues		
Mental health	Religious/spiritual beliefs	Relationship with healthcare staff	
Weight	Body image		
Diet	Previous experience		
Exercise	Trauma – past and present		
Smoking			
Alcohol/other substances	Stress		
Sleep	Coping style		
	Health behaviours		

← ——————————————————————— →

Data from Engel G.L. (1977).

symptoms of kidney disease (e.g. fatigue, nausea, restlessness, sleep difficulties, itching, anaemia), comorbid physical health problems, the awareness of decreased life expectancy and the impact of secondary factors resulting from having kidney disease (e.g. impact on family life, social life, work, financial concerns).

When considering the impact of CKD on a person, it is helpful to understand the multiple factors which can interact to affect a person's functioning (Table 5.1). Using a biopsychosocial approach can be useful to appreciate the interaction of biological, psychological (which includes thoughts, feelings and behaviour) and social factors, which can all play a significant role in the context of disease or illness (Engel 1977).

Why are psychosocial issues important?

Psychosocial issues are important not only in relation to maintaining a good quality of life. A growing body of evidence cites mental health as a predictor of patient outcomes in people with CKD (Hedayati *et al.* 2010, Tsai *et al.* 2012). People who have clinical depression prior to starting RRT have poorer outcomes and reduced long-term survival. This is likely to be in part related to the impact on health-related behaviours such as decreased self-care and reduced treatment concordance, but it may also be due to stress-mediated changes in physiological function. The National Institute for Health and Clinical Excellence (NICE) chronic kidney disease quality standard states that:

> People with established renal impairment should have access to psychosocial support (which may include support with personal, family, financial, employ-ment and/or social needs) appropriate to their circumstances (NICE 2011).

Increasingly, renal units have access to specialists such as clinical psychologists, counselling psychologists, health psychologists, counsellors and social workers, and they have an important role in supporting patients. However, the challenging psychosocial issues faced by people with CKD are common, and not all of these require specialist psychological intervention. It is important that psychosocial issues are understood by everyone who has a role in supporting the patient and that they are able to recognise distress and offer appropriate emotional and practical support, signposting and/or referring to other services as required.

Coping with diagnosis and encouraging acceptance

Receiving a diagnosis of CKD can be a difficult experience, and patients' responses can vary quite widely due to a number of factors. Some people have known about their kidney problems for a long time, and the progression of their condition and subsequent preparation for dialysis may be something they were expecting. However, it can still be shocking – they have been putting the possibility out of their mind and never believed it would happen to them. For those people unaware of having kidney problems, either because they have residual damage from an acute kidney injury or because they have received their diagnosis of CKD at stage 5, it can come as a significant shock.

People may find it difficult to become 'a patient' and particularly resent the loss of control they have over certain aspects of their care. Some people find inpatient hospital stays particularly difficult and resent the lack of privacy and the feelings of dependence on others.

Stages of acceptance

Patients will often go through a range of emotions as they accept their diagnosis, and it can be helpful to view this as a normal response to any loss or significant life event. People often go through a number of stages such as shock, denial, anger, bargaining, depression, and then work through their feelings and reach a stage of acceptance before moving on to plan for the future (Kübler-Ross 1969). Progress through these stages is not always strictly linear. It is beneficial to normalise how people are feeling about their diagnosis and to give them permission to talk and express their feelings. Listening and watchful waiting are helpful, as an adjustment reaction may progress into depression, particularly where people already have increased background risk factors (previous or current mental health issues, low social and family support, decreased activity or occupation). Patients who have an acute presentation of CKD and require an immediate start to dialysis are also at an increased risk of psychological difficulties. They have not had the educational, psychological and practical preparation and may require additional support to accept their condition.

Coping styles

A number of factors influence the way people cope with their illness. These include their personality, their beliefs about themselves, their condition, and their medical care. Self-efficacy, health locus of control and illness representations can also affect the way a person manages his or her health condition. For example, people who believe they are capable of managing their symptoms, take responsibility for their treatment and believe that people can live well with CKD, are likely to cope better and be less distressed.

In general, adjustment tends to improve over time, although some people adopt coping strategies that may not appear overtly helpful. For example, they may deny they are unwell or refuse to make a decision about treatment (Box 5.1). On one level, these strategies can actually be protective, enabling a person to continue with everyday life, but they can become counterproductive. When someone gets stuck with a particular emotion (e.g. anger) and refuses to engage with the medical team, or if a patient's behaviour is potentially harming his or her health, it may indicate a need for additional specialist support.

Encouraging self-management

Encouraging patients to self-manage their health issues will also help them to accept their condition (Table 5.2). There are a number of prerequisites to self-management, particularly access to information and the opportunity to be involved in shared decision making about care. Encouraging patients to access their blood test results, monitor their blood pressure at home, and engage in positive health-related behaviours can increase their personal sense of control over their condition. It can be difficult to influence health-related behaviour change if a person does not see that an issue exists – e.g. 'I don't have a problem with my diet.' Sometimes a patient will have a specific concern, and improvements in this area may encourage them to be more open to addressing other health-related issues and behaviour.

Box 5.1 Patient story: denial and acceptance

Sarah was referred to the renal unit and was diagnosed with CKD stage 5 following a medical assessment for a new job. It came as a complete shock to her and she reported that she did not feel unwell. She questioned the blood test results and felt that 'they must have made a mistake'. After a number of appointments with a pre-dialysis specialist nurse she agreed that she would have haemodialysis 'if the need arose' but refused to have a fistula for access. She then started to miss follow-up clinic appointments.

Sarah was referred to the renal counsellor and she agreed to attend. She talked about how hard it had been when her father died in hospital. She had always avoided hospital and was so scared that she would die that she could not even contemplate that the diagnosis could be true. Once she started to talk about her fears she became very distressed. Eventually she was able to re-engage with the medical team and agreed to the fistula creation. She continued to deny that she was feeling unwell until she started dialysis.

Sarah used denial to enable her to continue with everyday life and avoid feeling distress, but with support she was able to accept the need to prepare for treatment.

Table 5.2 Key points: coping and adjusting to life with CKD.

- Finding it difficult to adjust to a diagnosis may be a normal reaction. Patients should have the opportunity to talk about how they feel, and should be reassured that their responses are normal.
- People adjust differently to their diagnosis and treatment regimes. Those with a higher risk of adjustment difficulties may need specialist support.
- Supported self-management often improves patients' knowledge and willingness to self-care, as well as helping them to accept their condition and feel more in control.

Some patients find group programmes helpful. For example, programmes such as the Expert Patient Programme run over six weeks and include topics such as dealing with pain, tiredness, coping with depression, relaxation techniques, exercise, diet, communication and planning for the future. Although not specific to kidney disease, much of the material is appropriate and is available in face-to-face groups and online. (Note, however, that when encouraging patients to access general self-help materials it is important to warn them that dietary advice will not be specific to their condition and they should continue to follow the dietary advice of the renal team).

> ## Box 5.2   Patient story: improving self-management
>
> Peter had developed CKD stage 4 as a consequence of type 2 diabetes. He openly admitted that he had never managed his diabetes particularly well as he had never really accepted his condition. He found it difficult to talk about CKD and did not ask any questions in appointments with the medical team.
>
> When asked about his health concerns by his general practitioner, he said he wanted to lose some weight but because he was so tired he had reduced his physical activity and was not doing any exercise. He said he often forgot to take his blood pressure medication. His practice nurse explained he could still exercise, and he started to walk more and swim twice a week. He also started to monitor his blood pressure at home and his blood pressure medication concordance improved. Following improvements in his overall health, he asked his GP to refer him for self-management support to improve the control of his diabetes, and he started to engage more actively in his renal clinic appointments.

Fatigue is a significant symptom of CKD and often results in people reducing their physical activity levels (Box 5.2). This can become a vicious circle which leads to decreased physical and emotional health. The evidence supports the positive benefit of exercise on both physical and mental health, and referral to a community exercise programme to enable people to increase their regular activity may also be helpful (Heiwe & Jacobson 2011).

Impact on family, social life and work

Family life

CKD can have a significant impact on a person's family relationships. The strains of ill health and the demands of dialysis treatment (whether home or hospital-based) can negatively impact on family life. Social support, and particularly the support from a partner, has been shown to be a protective factor and is linked to increased quality of life and improved mental health. Those people without a partner may have concerns that their condition will adversely affect any future relationships. CKD can bring additional stress to current relationships as there may be significant changes to the roles people assume within the relationship. For example, a person with CKD may no longer be able to contribute to the family income or may find that their partner has become their carer. Their partner may have to take on additional activities at home (e.g. housework or childcare), and individuals may struggle with feeling dependent and a burden on their family (Box 5.3).

> ## Box 5.3 Patient story: family life and psychosexual difficulties
>
> Helen was married with one child and had recently had a transplant. She was finding it difficult to recover and felt guilty that her husband undertook the majority of the housework as well as working full-time. She also felt very guilty about the impact of her illness on her child and she worried about what would happen to her family if she died prematurely. She felt very unattractive because of her surgical scars and reported that she had not had sex in the last year, mainly because of tiredness. She said her husband was accepting of this but she was concerned that he would leave her for someone else. Her friends were mostly related to her previous employment and she rarely saw them any more. She generally spent most days at home watching TV and wished she could return to the 'person she was'.
>
> Helen's situation illustrates the complex relationship between psychological, social and physical problems. Helen agreed to see a counselling psychologist with her husband. The psychologist worked with her to increase her activity and to emotionally and cognitively accept the changes which had occurred. She talked about her fears for the future with her husband, and they engaged in some psychosexual therapy which improved their relationship. At discharge Helen had started some voluntary work and felt she was contributing more to their family life.

Home dialysis may offer an improved quality of life but may incur an additional burden on families, who may also need practical and emotional support. Health problems can limit a family's activities and impact on opportunities for holidays. It can be helpful to encourage families to continue with these activities where possible. It is important to emphasise that though it may take more planning, people with CKD are often still able to travel and should be encouraged to do so, as this provides a break for the family as well as themselves.

Patients with children sometimes struggle with changes in their parenting role. They may feel guilty about the impact of their health on their children, particularly if they have an acute admission. In some areas there are young carer support groups which provide additional help for children with a parent with CKD.

Sexual dysfunction is common in people with CKD, but patients often find it difficult to raise the subject with health professionals. Patients should be encouraged to broach the subject during appointments with their specialist team or general practitioner. Both men and women describe a number of problems including a decrease in sexual interest and impotence. It is likely that a combination of organic causes, treatment effects and psychosocial factors contribute to the aetiology of sexual dysfunction. It is important that underlying health causes are identified and patients are offered information, treatment options and psychosexual counselling if required.

Social support

Kidney disease can affect friendships and social relationships. People with CKD may be less able to engage in social activities and may find that friends do not understand the implications of their health condition or have unrealistic expectations. A number of people talk about finding it more difficult to go out because of increased fatigue, and find that fluid and dietary restrictions limit social activities such as eating out, leading to an increased sense of isolation. People value the support of their friends, and maintaining relationships can be very beneficial.

There is evidence that social support can act as a buffer against stressful events and also appears to impact on health outcomes including quality of life and treatment concordance. Social support has been linked to higher rates of survival in CKD, which underlines the important role it has (Cohen *et al.* 2007). There are a number of possible mechanisms to explain the role of social support, including improved perception of quality of life and improved concordance with treatment. Patients can benefit from peer support from other people with CKD, and some renal units are developing more formal approaches to training for peer support volunteers.

Work and activity

Work and activity is beneficial for both emotional and physical wellbeing (Waddell & Burton 2006). Work provides structure to a day and increases social interaction, and in addition to financial benefits it can also improve self-esteem and confidence. Many people with CKD work full-time, but this may come at a cost, with limited energy for other family and social activities. Unfortunately people with CKD can find it difficult to continue working in their current role due to periods of ill health or high levels of fatigue. A person who is struggling with work needs to be realistic about the type of work and the hours they can cope with. This is particularly an issue where people are trying to maintain work around dialysis treatment. People with CKD may not view themselves as 'disabled' and will often be unaware that they are protected in law from discrimination in the workplace. Employers should make reasonable adjustments for the needs of people with CKD, although often both employers and employees are unaware of the options available to help someone to continue working. Depending on the circumstances, there may be opportunities for part-time work, flexible start and finish times, job-sharing, home working or self-employment. People are often anxious about raising their health problems with their employers and may need support and encouragement to do so. Additional support and advice on the options for staying in work and the benefit entitlements for those leaving work can be accessed via a renal social worker, a disability employment adviser based in a job centre or through welfare rights services.

Stopping work through ill health or retirement can bring about significant social and psychological changes, and it can be helpful to encourage people to adopt or maintain activities through which to structure their day. Hobbies and activities may need to change to accommodate physical and practical

> ## Box 5.4 Patient story: the impact of work and social activities
>
> Peter started on continuous ambulatory peritoneal dialysis (CAPD) and had recently stopped working because of his health problems. He used to have a very active social life mainly orientated around the pub. Since starting CAPD he had stopped going out as he couldn't drink as he had before. He was very concerned about his finances and worried that he couldn't pay the bills.
>
> Peter was referred to see a social worker, who assisted him with making applications for benefits and encouraged him to engage in more activity, and he decided to start gardening at an allotment. He joined a gardening group and returned to part-time work. At a follow-up appointment, Peter was socially very busy at weekends and he was considering increasing his hours at work.
>
> This example highlights how important social relationships, activity and work are in contributing to a person's sense of motivation and wellbeing.

limitations. Some people may reluctantly have to reduce or stop the activities they are unable to participate in and may need support and encouragement to develop new interests. Educational courses, retraining and voluntary work offer opportunities to maintain activity and develop new skills (Box 5.4).

Financial issues

Changes in health often impact on a person's financial situation. Older people may express concerns about applying for support and feel that they do not deserve help. Some people will not have any experience of applying for state benefits, and they may need support from a renal social worker or signposting to welfare rights services which can help with their applications. Patients do not always qualify for, or may be refused, support, and in these circumstances specialist welfare advice may be able to assist. People who have significant social care needs can request an assessment from social services both for themselves and for their carer.

Young adults with CKD

Young adults with CKD have been identified as a vulnerable group at risk of poor treatment outcomes. There has been increased recognition that having CKD as a young adult impacts greatly on many areas of life, including education, employment and relationships (Box 5.5). Coping with kidney disease may impact on the social development of young adults and interfere with their progression through the normal developmental stages of adolescence. Some young adults will be faced with leaving the relative security of a paediatric service and transitioning to an adult service where they will become aware

Box 5.5   Patient story: supporting young adults with kidney disease

Basim was diagnosed with CKD stage 5 at age 17. He transferred from paediatric services to the adult renal unit just as he started dialysis treatment (CAPD). He had a good attendance record in paediatrics but often missed appointments in the adult unit. He said he was too busy to make appointments to see his specialist nurse, and staff were concerned that he was not adhering to his treatment schedule. At his next clinic appointment his kidney consultant broached the subject with him. He said he was undertaking his treatment but he found it very difficult to fit it around his apprentice job and he was anxious about taking any time off work. He said he found it difficult to remember appointments and it had been easier when his mother had organised everything for him. He felt very alone, because no one else in his circle of friends had CKD.

Basim is an example of a young man who is struggling to adjust to living with and self-managing a chronic health condition. He is feeling socially isolated and is finding it very difficult to access support. Basim would particularly benefit from services targeted at young adults, and from opportunities to meet other young people with CKD. He needs support to develop the skills to enable him to manage his current treatment and increase the likelihood that he will be concordant with future treatment options, e.g. a transplant.

Table 5.3   Key points: impact on family, social life and work.

- CKD can have a significant impact on family relationships. Family carers may need additional practical and emotional support.
- Sexual dysfunction is common and can have a negative impact on relationships. Patients can find it difficult to broach and discuss these issues.
- Maintaining social relationships, and continuing work and social activities, contributes to a person's sense of wellbeing.
- Young adults with CKD can be a vulnerable group and may require increased support to encourage independent living skills, develop social relationships and access work opportunities.

that they are different in age to the majority of the adult renal population. Young adults who present to the adult service for the first time with CKD have to adjust to their diagnosis and treatment as well as assess the impact on their life plans. Although young adults with CKD are a small population they may need specialist psychosocial support with a wide range of emotional and practical issues. For example, a young person who is finding it difficult to manage their own medication after a transplant could potentially lose their graft if they are not supported to better manage their treatment (Table 5.3).

Coping with dialysis treatment

Coping with dialysis treatment can be stressful. A number of factors appear to affect a patient's ability to adapt to treatment, including their coping style, social support, length of time on dialysis and previous and current mental health issues. Patients will often describe a number of difficult psychosocial issues, and several will be considered here.

Treatment choices – home versus hospital treatment

Patients with CKD are asked to make decisions about the type and location of treatment. Pre-dialysis education is essential to empower patients to make informed decisions; however, people use different strategies to make decisions and may need support to review the available options. The views of other people (e.g. friends, family, other patients) may influence a person's decision. It is helpful to encourage people to take time over making a decision and to ask about how they have come to decisions in the past for clues as to a person's decision-making style. It is useful to talk about a person's values – what is particularly important to them? We can also assist reasoning with decision aids, which are resources that help patients to fully consider their situation and make choices between the available treatment options.

There is some evidence to suggest that those undertaking peritoneal dialysis (PD) and home haemodialysis experience greater wellbeing and less distress than those undertaking hospital dialysis (Cameron *et al.* 2000). However, this may also relate to patient bias in the evidence, since younger and healthier

---

Box 5.6   Patient story: supporting choices and transitions in care

Adam was treated by hospital dialysis three times a week. He had multiple health problems including diabetes, an amputation and visual impairment. Adam lived with his wife, who was his main carer and accompanied him when he attended hospital. Adam told his consultant that he was thinking about stopping treatment as he hated the travelling time and having to leave the house for his regular dialysis – it felt like 'too much effort'.

Adam initially refused to consider a home-based therapy, but eventually he and his wife both agreed to try the option. Training occurred very quickly, as Adam's wife was already aware of many practical aspects of his treatment. Once they were at home Adam was able to have shorter, more frequent dialysis, and he saw improved health benefits from this. The practical demands on Adam's wife increased, but they agreed to access some regular respite care for Adam. Adam felt much more in control of his treatment and decided to continue with treatment at home.

patients are more likely to choose a home-based therapy. Dialysing at home allows greater treatment flexibility but is associated with increased responsibility and practical demands on the person and their family. For some people a hospital-based therapy may allow them to separate their illness from the rest of their life, whereas for others the inflexibility of a hospital-based therapy has a negative psychosocial impact. It is important that people are enabled to make informed choices, as this improves their personal sense of control over their treatment (Box 5.6).

Time

Whichever treatment modality (hospital or home haemodialysis, continuous or automated peritoneal dialysis) is chosen, it involves time. Prior to starting treatment people may underestimate this and hope they will fit it in around their other commitments. While it is important for patients to continue their everyday activities, trying to fit everything in around dialysis sessions is likely to be difficult, and sometimes impossible. People often resent travelling and/ or treatment preparation time, and they typically find treatment boring. For example, a person on automated peritoneal dialysis (APD) may resent having to be at home to complete their 10-hour treatment session overnight, which is usually prescribed for at least six nights a week. A person on hospital dialysis may resent the long travelling time.

Concordance issues

People particularly complain about fluid and dietary restrictions and the negative impact that these have on the quality of their life. This can lead to poor dietary and fluid concordance. People may also have difficulties with taking medication. A number of people have difficulties maintaining concordance with treatment schedules for a number of reasons including the time treatment takes and the frequency of dialysis. Non-concordance is a complex issue and can lead to poor health outcomes. It may relate to the lack of acceptance of their diagnosis or to a wider pattern of non-adherence in other areas of their lives.

A number of strategies can be used where non-concordance is an issue. Staff can support patient understanding of the issues through education. Exploring specific patient concerns and working cooperatively to address these issues is helpful. Some individuals may need more frequent support, and may benefit from continuity with the same staff members. It is important to respond positively to small improvements in concordance and not to underestimate the work it can take to change habitual behaviour (Box 5.7).

Needle phobia and traumatic experiences

Needle phobia is not an uncommon difficulty amongst dialysis patients, which may be related to previous negative experiences of needle procedures. It unfortunately may limit a patient's choice of treatment and cause clinic

> ## Box 5.7 Patient story: improving concordance with treatment
>
> Safeerah had been coming for hospital dialysis for six months. Initially she had adjusted well to dialysis but over the last few months she had become increasingly withdrawn. Staff noticed that she appeared very unhappy and did not speak to anyone unless she was asked a question. She started to miss dialysis sessions.
>
> Her primary nurse took some time to talk to her about her difficulties, and Safeerah talked about how much she hated the time sitting on dialysis. She felt as if it was wasted time. The unit had an exercise-on-dialysis programme, and the nurse encouraged Safeerah to take part in this. Initially Safeerah was quite self-conscious and needed some support and encouragement from the staff team. She started to enjoy her exercise sessions and said that she felt she was doing something useful with her time. The nurse also suggested some other activities for her to engage in while she was on dialysis. Safeerah had moderate visual impairment and found reading difficult but decided that she would access audio books via the library.
>
> A combination of exercise and engaging in an enjoyable activity changed the way in which Safeerah viewed dialysis, and her attendance increased. Her mood improved and she started to interact more with staff and patients on the unit.

appointments and blood tests to become stressful. It is important to distinguish between a fear of needles and a blood phobia. Needle phobia will often result in increased anxiety and an increase in blood pressure, in contrast to blood phobia, which results in a sudden decrease in blood pressure and can lead to the person fainting. In some people needle exposure alone can also trigger an anticipatory blood pressure drop which can cause fainting. These difficulties require specialist psychological intervention with different treatment approaches.

Given the seriousness of the condition and its treatment over years, it is not uncommon for patients with CKD to experience or witness traumatic events which can have an immediate or cumulative effect – for example, being in Intensive care, experiencing painful or difficult medical procedures, seeing other patients become unwell and unfortunately sometimes witnessing the death of their peers. These experiences may result in post-traumatic symptoms which may improve over time. It is helpful to encourage people to talk to their friends and family. Symptoms which do not improve may benefit from further psychological intervention (Box 5.8).

Body image

Body image is not a static concept, and it is influenced by many factors including personal experience, personality, society and culture. A person's

Box 5.8   Patient story: needle phobia and supporting self-care

Lily was currently undertaking PD but she had been told that she would need to transfer to HD for medical reasons. Lily had chosen to have PD as she had severe fear of needles and she could not imagine undertaking a therapy involving them.

Lily was referred to a clinical psychologist for assessment and intervention. Lily could relate her fear of needles to an experience when she was a small child and she had been held down by two staff members who had been unable to place a cannula in her hand. With the psychologist she worked on managing her anxiety, using specific cognitive and behavioural techniques. Using a structured graded process, she was gradually exposed to needles and she was able to look at and touch needles and to watch other people having needles inserted for dialysis.

When Lily started haemodialysis, the nurses on the unit supported her to become self-caring, and using the techniques she had learned to manage her anxiety she found that she could cope better if she was able to put in her own needles. Subsequently she decided to train for home HD therapy, which was something she had never considered possible.

Table 5.4   Key points: supporting acceptance, choice and self-management.

- Information and support with decision making enables people to choose treatment that fits with their lifestyle.
- Whichever treatment modality is chosen for dialysis, treatment takes time and people may need support to adjust to this change.
- People may struggle with treatment, fluid and dietary concordance. People may need ongoing support to make changes in this area.
- Both needle phobia and the impact of traumatic medical experiences can be improved with specialist psychological support.
- Treatment for CKD may result in changes to a person's body image, and this may impact on interpersonal relationships and treatment decisions.

perception of their appearance can be different from how others actually perceive them. There are a number of changes which can occur due to CKD. For example fistula formation, PD tube insertion and surgical scarring are all common. People with a visible difference have less choice about disclosure than those with differences that are either invisible or a combination of visible and invisible. As in Helen's story (Box 5.3), body image issues amongst patients with CKD can have an impact on relationships and sexual functioning (Table 5.4). Other people may be reluctant to have particular procedures (e.g. fistula formation) because of concerns about the impact on physical appearance.

People may use different strategies to cope with visible differences: including choosing to actively disclose their condition or attempting to conceal it and changing their behaviour or avoiding specific situations to reduce the possibility of people discovering the difference. Where body image issues are having a negative impact on a person's day-to-day functioning, that person may benefit from more specialist psychological support.

Transplant issues

There is agreement that kidney transplantation is the best treatment in suitable patients, but there are a number of psychosocial issues relating to receiving a transplant that can make it a complex area and potentially an emotional rollercoaster. Attitudes toward transplantation differ with age, background and personality. Some people find it difficult to accept the concept of receiving a kidney donation at all. Although many people are able to accept a transplant from a deceased donor, some people continue to struggle to come to terms with the fact that a person has died. In these situations, anniversaries and special occasions may become distressing reminders for recipients of a transplant.

Some people have similar reservations in accepting a kidney from a living related donor. For example, some people talk about the natural order of donation – parents donate to children and not the other way around. Living related donations can also be complicated where family relationships are strained or people are not altruistically motivated to donate. For example, they may feel they have to, or may feel guilty because they do not want to do it. Both donors and recipients may find it difficult to express their doubts or concerns. Specialist kidney services often involve a psychologist or a psychiatrist to provide a psychological assessment prior to transplantation. Where potential living donors do not offer to donate a kidney this can also cause a person distress. However, it is also worth noting that living related donation is often successful and can strengthen interpersonal relationships.

Waiting – life on the list

Waiting for a deceased-donor transplant can extend over several years and inevitably means living with constant uncertainty. People may use a number of coping strategies to manage this time, including denial ('it will never happen'), social support, and rationalisation ('it will happen at some point but I can't put my life on hold'). When the call that notifies the patient of a potential donor actually comes, its unexpectedness can lead to a range of emotions including surprise, excitement and fear. People may also find it difficult if the transplant does not go ahead (usually due to positive cross-match or inter-current illness, or because they have been called in as a reserve candidate), particularly if they have received a number of previous calls.

Adjustment after transplant

Following a transplant, some people can struggle emotionally if the graft does not immediately work, and this can become difficult if the graft does not function at all. It is an unpredictable situation in which they have a loss of control over the outcome. If the graft functions, people may also struggle to adjust to the new routine of appointments and a different treatment regime. People who attended hospital dialysis may miss their fellow patients. A number of people find it difficult to make the necessary changes to their diet and fluid intake, particularly where they had tightly controlled limits due to dialysis. Although people are never told that transplantation is a 'cure', people can implicitly believe that it will return their life to how it was before they were unwell. Patients can therefore feel disappointed when they do not return to their previous level of functioning, and this potentially may precipitate depression.

Some people experience significant anxiety symptoms post transplant and fear that something will go wrong. They may become obsessive in relation to taking care of their health and limit their engagement in activities. It can be helpful to support them to recognise that the transplant may not last until the end of their life but that they can enjoy the opportunity and lifestyle freedom it gives them.

Adjustment to life post transplant may also impact on medication concordance. Early non-concordance with transplant medication appears to predict poorer longer-term outcomes. This can be a problem where the person is finding it difficult to adjust to body image changes post transplant (including surgical scars, changes to body shape and steroid-induced changes), which can be accentuated further by their medication. If anxiety or adjustment difficulties are severe, specialist support may be helpfully offered.

Transplant loss

There are a number of emotions and practical issues that occur when people are told that their graft is failing. For some people it can be a shock, even when it has been happening over a period of time. They may have experienced previous episodes of rejection with better outcomes and not have anticipated a negative outcome. A range of specialist staff are experienced in preparing potential kidney recipients for the possibility of a deterioration in the functioning of a transplant, but patients may have avoided thinking about the eventual loss and may experience a significant shock when it happens. Ideally they will have had some time to come to terms with the change in treatment, but unfortunately that is not always the case. We often use terminology such as 'failed transplant', and this in itself can be seen as value-ridden. People can feel guilty at the loss of the transplant, and this can be further intensified if the cause of the graft loss was related to non-concordance with treatment. Some people experience a bereavement reaction in response to the loss. Where the donor was living-related the person may also feel additional guilt over the impact of the graft loss on the donor.

For those who have experienced dialysis before, returning to dialysis can pose a number of problems. Those who have experienced difficulties on dialysis may also struggle (Box 5.9). Patients who have received pre-emptive transplants will be faced with the same issues as someone approaching dialysis for the first time, and it is important that they receive the same pre-dialysis

---

Box 5.9   Patient story: anxiety, loss and adjustment

At the age of 49, John was referred for counselling shortly after he had received a live-donor transplant from his sister. This was his second transplant. The first transplant, from a deceased donor, had lasted for 18 years. He expressed strong sadness about the loss of his first transplant and the deceased donor. He felt he had no opportunity to express these feelings of loss, which were in turn linked to an increased awareness of his own mortality. He said that he did not want anything to happen to this kidney because it was his sister's gift. He spent a long time worrying about the future and found it very difficult to contemplate having to go back to dialysis treatment in the future. He felt extremely anxious about his new kidney and felt he had to engage in checking behaviour to ensure nothing was going wrong. This meant that he would check his computer test results every day to reassure himself that his kidney function was OK even though he knew logically that there were no new results to see. He found it very difficult to leave the house, as he was concerned that he might pick up an infection or have an accident and damage the kidney.

This is an example of somebody who had not yet come to terms with the loss of his first kidney. His fears for the future were stopping him taking the opportunity he currently had to improve the quality of his life. John was engaging in a number of behaviours, e.g. checking and not going out, which he thought were helping him feel better but were actually increasing his anxiety.

Table 5.5   Key points: issues around transplantation.

- Transplantation is a complex area. There are many psychosocial factors relating to the acceptance of being a donor or recipient.
- Waiting for a transplant can be a difficult time, and people may be unprepared when the call comes.
- People may find it difficult to adjust after receiving a transplant. They may have increased anxiety, or may be unhappy if their expectations are not realised.
- Graft loss can be experienced as a significant loss, and people may need support to adjust to dialysis treatment.

education and counselling which they would have received in a pre-dialysis clinic setting. This group of patients may have increased difficulty adjusting to dialysis, because they are coping with a new treatment as well as the loss of their transplant (Table 5.5).

End-of-life issues

For most people a 'good death' is one which occurs in their chosen location, with the people they want there, where they are comfortable, their physical, emotional and spiritual needs are met, and life is not unnecessarily prolonged (Smith 2000). Unfortunately we do not always fulfil a person's wishes for their end-of-life care. Most people, when asked, would prefer to die at home – but the majority die in hospital (Leadbeater & Garber 2010).

In general, both patients and staff often struggle to talk about death (Box 5.10). Patients can feel very anxious about things but are unable to express their concerns. Families may also avoid talking about death, as they want to focus on the person staying alive. This can leave the person feeling anxious and unable to discuss their fears for the future. It can leave staff struggling to meet the psychosocial needs of the patient. This is particularly important in cases where conservative treatment options may offer the patient improved quality of life.

**Box 5.10   Patient story: supporting patients
to discuss their death anxieties**

Mary's health had been rapidly deteriorating over the last six months, and staff on the unit had noticed that she appeared to be low in mood. Mary talked with staff about how she was really scared about dying. It was arranged for Mary to meet with the renal palliative care nurse. Mary was able to explain that although she recognised that she would probably die in the next year her fear was around the actual process of dying. She had heard from another patient that 'some renal patients died from drowning in their own fluid if they stop dialysis' and this had scared her. She had tried to talk to her son about her concerns but he had said that she was being silly and that she was not likely to die any time soon. Mary found it extremely helpful to be given some information about end-of-life care for people with kidney disease, and she decided she would like to document her wishes for her future care.

Mary benefited from information which helped settle her anxiety, and she found it supportive to talk to somebody outside her family about the issues. Following her discussions with the staff she was able to talk to her family about her concerns and her wishes for future care.

Parents and grandparents

End-of-life issues are particularly difficult when the person with CKD has children or grandchildren who are under 18. Children may be affected by the serious illness of their parent/grandparent. Supporting parents/grandparents with CKD to make plans for the end of their life is helpful. They may require additional support to think about how they are going to talk to their children/grandchildren about the issues. There are a number of books and resources available and it can be helpful to encourage people to create memory boxes for their children/grandchildren before they die.

Death anxiety

People typically fear the dying process and are frightened that they will lose control. Providing information and enabling people to discuss their wishes helps them exercise some level of control over their future care. Some staff can find it difficult to broach the subject of death, and not everyone is ready to have these conversations. The timing needs to take into account the person's current needs and whether they are receptive to discussing their situation. It can be helpful to ask a person if they have any concerns about their future, as this may give them the opportunity to talk about their worries. It is also useful to explain why you are raising the issue, particularly where death is not imminent. Hearing about other people's experiences of death and the options, such as treatment choices which may be available, can be helpful. It is important that the conversation focuses on listening to the person and not just on providing information or making future plans.

Withdrawal from dialysis

Withdrawal from dialysis usually occurs where there is no benefit in further prolonging a person's life – such as when the patient is dying or when quality of life is reduced to such an extent that there is no expectation it can be improved. People will sometimes request withdrawal from dialysis, and in other situations the person decides they have 'had enough' of treatment. There is evidence to suggest that this is linked to an increased level of clinical depression (McDade-Montez *et al*. 2006). It is important in these cases to explore reasons for withdrawal, particularly to identify any factors which might be temporary or might respond to appropriate interventions, e.g. mental distress, physical pain, unhappiness with the treatment modality, social care needs and availability of family and social support. In these situations a person may be willing to postpone a decision to withdraw from dialysis to enable potential changes and additional support to be put in place to improve their quality of life. These are difficult circumstances, and specialist advice and support is usually indicated (Table 5.6).

Table 5.6 Key points: issues around death and dying.

- For most people a 'good death' is one which supports their physical, psychological and spiritual needs.
- Patients, families and staff can all find it difficult to talk about death.
- It can be helpful to provide opportunities for people to talk about their fears.
- The wish to withdraw from dialysis treatment can be associated with depression, and it is useful to consider the factors which are potentially changeable and can improve a person's quality of life.
- Parents and grandparents with CKD may need support not only to plan for the end of their own life but also to support their children or grandchildren.

Specialist support services

There is a general role for all staff in both primary and secondary care to support people with CKD (Box 5.11). There is often a desire on the part of the professional to provide practical help with problems, and as this chapter has shown there are many different opportunities to do this. However, several of the psychosocial challenges faced by patients with CKD do not have a solution. In these situations it is sometimes easier for the professional to avoid the topic and not discuss the issues. People with chronic, life-limiting conditions often gain comfort and reassurance from professionals who are willing to listen and show compassion and concern. People with CKD often build close relationships with staff over an extended period of time, and these are a source of ongoing support. Communicating in a sensitive way, using advanced listening skills, giving people the opportunity to talk about their feelings and acknowledging these is very beneficial and should not be overlooked in favour of a referral to a specialist practitioner.

One of the practical challenges staff face is in differentiating whether a person's distress is a normal response to a difficult and stressful set of circumstances or evidence of more significant mental health issues which could benefit from more active support and treatment. There are a number of screening instruments available which can indicate distress, and distinguish between states such as anxiety, depression and obsessive compulsive disorder. It is important that these are used alongside talking to the person about their difficulties and needs. For those people with continuing levels of distress, further psychological intervention may be required. People can find it difficult to accept the suggestion that they could benefit from a referral for specialist support for their psychological problems, and staff should raise the issue with sensitivity and gain consent before referring a patient to a specialist professional.

Box 5.11 Patient story: psychological therapy to work with depression

William has a diagnosis of polycystic kidney disease and has had treatment for over 20 years. He had been waiting on the national list for six years for a potential third transplant. He was currently on hospital haemodialysis when he was first referred to the renal clinical psychologist for depression, and his presentation suggested that significant symptoms were present. He was finding it difficult to get to sleep and was waking very early in the morning. He reported finding it difficult to motivate himself to do things and that he was increasingly tearful. He had had thoughts that he would be 'better off dead' but did not plan to do anything to harm himself as he did not want to hurt his wife.

He did not want to take another tablet and initially did not want to take antidepressants. However, his GP encouraged him to start antidepressant medication and William agreed to engage in psychological therapy. Using a cognitive behavioural approach, the clinical psychologist was able to work with William to increase his day-to-day activity and to set realistic goals to improve his quality of life. William was able to modify his thoughts about his illness and no longer saw himself as a burden. The psychologist also taught William to use mindfulness to enable him to recognise the patterns of thinking and feelings that were increasing his distress. This approach encouraged him to become more compassionate to himself and to change these patterns. William reported that he was feeling better and was increasingly able to cope with his chronic health problems. Working with his GP, he felt able to stop the antidepressant medication and he continued to use mindfulness to support himself.

Referring to specialist services

Renal services often have a number of other specialists working within the team, including psychologists, counsellors and social workers. They also work closely with services such as mental health. Although there are similarities in the way these professionals work, it is important to recognise that the roles are not interchangeable and each professional works in a different way to support patients and/or alleviate psychological distress. The advantage of specialists based within the renal team is that they are in a better position to offer intervention which takes into account the impact of CKD, and they also work collaboratively within the team. As well as support from specialist workers, individuals who may benefit from psychotropic medication often require primary care and/or secondary mental health support. There is a useful role for medication in those people with more significant mental health problems. Those with severe and enduring mental health problems are likely to need long-term services from community mental health and/or social care. For those patients experiencing an acute mental health crisis, it is important that support is accessed from secondary mental health support or mental health crisis services, as most renal psychologists, counsellors and social workers are not resourced or equipped to respond to an acute mental health crisis.

Provision for specialist services varies in different areas. Where renal services do not have a specialist worker available, referrals to other services can be made through the patient's general practitioner. Acute hospitals may also have access to psychiatric liaison or psychological medicine, who may accept referrals depending on their service specifications. High rates of depression can lead to an increased risk of suicidal ideation and suicide, and it is helpful for all staff to be familiar with evaluating mental health risk and the local referral pathways to access mental health crisis services (Keskin & Engin 2011).

Psychological therapy/counselling

NICE recommends the use of cognitive behavioural therapy (CBT) for people with depression and anxiety, and there is growing evidence for CBT within a renal context as an individual and group intervention for depression (Hedayati et al. 2012), and specifically to improve fluid concordance (Sharp et al. 2005) and sleep disturbance (Chen et al. 2008). However, the psychological difficulties a person with CKD may have when referred may be more complex. A number of different therapeutic approaches may be beneficial, and these include but are not limited to CBT (e.g. behavioural therapy, person-centred counselling, motivational interviewing, couple and family work). Individuals should receive an assessment which enables an understanding of the nature and causes of their current difficulties and can enable the most appropriate intervention to be identified. Newer therapeutic approaches (e.g. mindfulness, acceptance and commitment therapy and compassion-focused therapy) show particular promise in helping patients to accept and adjust to their condition. All staff have a role in supporting psychological therapy, and multidisciplinary working can be helpful to the patient, the family and staff (Table 5.7).

Table 5.7 Key points: general and specialist support.

- Staff from both primary and secondary care have an important role in supporting people with CKD with their psychological issues.
- Supportive listening is very helpful, particularly where problems cannot be easily solved.
- The renal service may include a number of different professionals who can provide specialist psychological support. Support can also be accessed from local primary and secondary mental health services.
- Psychological therapy and/or medication have been successfully used to support people with CKD who have psychological difficulties.

Hope

There are many potential psychological and social consequences of CKD, and these can be easily viewed as a long list of negative experiences. However, hope has been shown to be an independent predictor of adjustment for people with CKD (Billington *et al.* 2008). All staff can actively support people with CKD to maintain appropriate hopefulness alongside the psychosocial issues that they encounter.

Adversity can lead to growth, and many individuals can experience positive change through adversity. People are extremely resilient, and our role is to not just to support the person with a particular difficult issue but to help them build their resilience and coping skills to enable them to take the next steps to the rest of their lives.

Conclusion: patient journeys

You can't stop the waves, but you can learn to surf (Kabat-Zinn 2004).

When a person develops CKD, they already have a background history which will impact on how they adjust to their condition. In addition, during the trajectory of their illness, they will experience a wide and varying range of physical, psychological and social issues. There are many points of transition, such as becoming a patient, transferring from paediatric to adult services, commencing RRT, receiving a transplant, returning to RRT and following an end-of-life pathway. These are likely to be times of psychological and social change, and increased stress for the patient is to be expected. Unresolved adjustment difficulties at these times can lead to more significant longer-term problems which may have a negative impact on a person's physical, mental and social functioning. Early intervention is important and can prevent longer-term difficulties. It is helpful for all staff to be aware of potential psychosocial issues and recognise when patients would benefit from additional support.

The nature and longevity of CKD means that patients and their families often have strong ties with the specialist team, and this can be a great source of comfort. Support for patients, their families and carers can take several forms. For many people, just discussing their concerns with someone who is actively listening can be helpful. For others, more active signposting or referral to specialist services within the community, primary care or renal services is important. Many of the issues the person will face on their renal journey are fixed – we cannot, for example, change the need for RRT or a transplant. However, with increased awareness of psychosocial issues, we can improve the direct support and psychological care we provide to enable people to live well with CKD.

Author's note

To maintain patient confidentiality, each of the patient stories is based on an amalgamation of different people's experiences and does not relate to any one specific individual.

References

Billington, E., Simpson, J., Unwin, J., Bray, D. & Giles, D. (2008) Does hope predict adjustment to end-stage renal failure and consequent dialysis? *British Journal of Health Psychology*, **13**, 683-99.

Cameron, J.I., Whiteside, C., Katz, J. & Devins, G.M. (2000) Differences in quality of life across renal replacement therapies: a meta-analytic comparison. *American Journal of Kidney Diseases*, **35**, 629-37.

Chen, H.Y., Chiang, C.K., Wang, H.H. *et al.* (2008) Cognitive-behavioral therapy for sleep disturbance in patients undergoing peritoneal dialysis: a pilot randomized controlled trial. *American Journal of Kidney Diseases*, **52**, 314-23.

Cohen, S.D., Sharma T., Acquaviv, K *et al.* (2007) Social support and chronic kidney disease: an update. *Advances in Chronic Kidney Disease*, **14**, 335-44.

Engel G.L. (1977) The need for a new medical model: a challenge for biomedicine. *Science*, **196**, 129-36.

Hedayati, S., Minhajuddin, A.T., Afshar, M. *et al.* (2010) Association between major depressive episodes in patients with chronic kidney disease and initiation of dialysis, hospitalization, or death. *JAMA*, **303**, 1946-53.

Hedayati, S.S., Yalamanchili, V. & Finkelstein, F.O. (2012) A practical approach to the treatment of depression in patients with chronic kidney disease and end-stage renal disease. *Kidney International*, **81**, 247-55.

Heiwe, S. & Jacobson, S.H. (2011) Exercise training for adults with chronic kidney disease. *Cochrane Database of Systematic Reviews*, (10), CD003236.

Kabat-Zinn, J. (2004) *Wherever You Go, There You Are*. Piatkus, London.

Keskin, G. & Engin, E. (2011) The evaluation of depression, suicidal ideation and coping strategies in haemodialysis patients with renal failure. *Journal of Clinical Nursing*, **20**, 2721-32.

Kübler-Ross, E. (1969) *On Death and Dying*. Routledge, London.

Leadbeater, C. & Garber, J. (2010) *Dying for Change*. Demos, London.

McDade-Montez, E.A., Christensen, A.J., Cvengros, J.A. & Lawton, W.J. (2006) The role of depression symptoms in dialysis withdrawal. *Health Psychology*, **25**, 198-204.

NICE (2009) *Depression in adults with a chronic physical health problem*. Treatment and management. National Institute for Health and Clinical Excellence, London.

NICE (2011) *Quality standard for chronic kidney disease in adults*. National Institute for Health and Clinical Excellence, London.

Sharp, J., Wild, M.R., Gumley, A.I. & Deighan, C.J. (2005) A cognitive behavioral group approach to enhance adherence to hemodialysis fluid restrictions: a randomized controlled trial. *American Journal of Kidney Diseases*, **45**, 1046-57.

Smith, R. (2000) A good death. *BMJ*, **320**, 129-30.

Tsai, Y.C., Chiu, Y.W., Hung, C.C. *et al.* (2012) Association of symptoms of depression with progression of CKD. *American Journal of Kidney Diseases*, **60**, 54-61.

Ver Halen, N., Cukor, D., Constantiner, M. & Kimmel, P. (2012) Depression and mortality in end-stage renal disease. *Current Psychiatry Reports*, **14**, 36-44.

Waddell, G. & Burton, A.K. (2006) *Is Work Good for Your Health and Well-Being?* The Stationery Office, London.

Watnick, S., Kirwin, P., Mahnensmith, R. & Concato, J (2003) The prevalence and treatment of depression among patients starting dialysis. *American Journal of Kidney Diseases*, **41**, 105-10.

Resources

Dying Matters is a broad-based and inclusive national coalition of nearly 17 000 members, which aims to change public knowledge, attitudes and behaviours towards death, dying and bereavement. http://www.dyingmatters.org (accessed September 2012).

Expert Patients Programme provide and deliver free courses aimed at helping people who are living with a long-term health condition to manage their condition better on a daily basis. http://www.expertpatients.co.uk (accessed September 2012).

The National Kidney Federation is the kidney patient charity in the UK, and aims to promote the best renal medical practice and treatment. The NKF also supports the needs of relatives and friends who care for kidney patients. The website provides useful information on a wide range of issues including medical and social issues, e.g. benefits and holidays. http://www.kidney.org.uk (accessed September 2012).

Winston's Wish is the leading childhood bereavement charity and the largest provider of services to bereaved children, young people and their families in the UK. http://www.winstonswish.org.uk (accessed September 2012).

Chapter 6

Acute Kidney Injury in Hospitalised Patients

Keith Harkins[1], Rachel Lewis[2] and Rachel Hilton[3]

[1]University Hospital of South Manchester, Manchester, UK
[2]Manchester Business School, The University of Manchester, UK
[3]Guy's and St Thomas' NHS Foundation Trust, London, UK

Introduction

Irrespective of the specialty, all hospitalised patients are at risk of acute kidney injury (AKI), which is associated with high levels of morbidity and mortality. The main purpose of this chapter is to provide a guide to assist in the diagnosis, management and prevention of AKI in hospitalised patients. AKI accounts for 1% of all hospital admissions and complicates 7% of inpatient episodes. Whilst the general principles of AKI management apply to a wider population, as the incidence is highest in older people this chapter focuses on managing AKI in an ageing population and includes some of the challenges particular to this cohort of patients.

What is 'elderly'?

This is not easy to define. When the first old age pensions were introduced by Lloyd George at the beginning of the last century, 'elderly' described those people who were too old to work. As the population has aged and the pension age has remained roughly the same, there is an expanding number of retired people. The proportion of retired people in the UK has increased from around 6% in 1901 to 17% (10.3 million people) today. Many of those who are in their sixties are now thought of as 'young old', and for the purposes of health care are not generally treated any differently from the rest of the adult population. There are, however, significant numbers of people who graduate into old age with one or more chronic conditions, and over recent years there has been an increase in those who live into extreme old age and become frail. It is predicted that the

Kidney Disease Management: A Practical Approach for the Non-Specialist Healthcare Practitioner, First Edition. Edited by Rachel Lewis and Helen Noble.
© 2013 John Wiley & Sons, Ltd. Published 2013 by John Wiley & Sons, Ltd.

proportion of elderly people in our society will continue to grow over the next 30 years, and that this increase will be in those living into their nineties and beyond.

'Frail' is a term often associated with the elderly, and most people have an idea of what it means. Frailty covers a spectrum of subjective meanings and there is no generic definition that can be applied to any one individual. Measuring frailty is difficult. There are over 20 different scales which generally measure physical factors such as diminishing nutritional status, physical activity, mobility, strength and energy, psychological aspects such as deteriorating cognition and mood, and social dimensions such as lack of social contacts and social support. The main difference in managing older adults compared to younger ones is the need to take account of the degree of frailty that occurs due to the physiological changes associated with advancing age and the accumulation of disease that often accompanies it.

Physiology of ageing

Most people would be able to describe the physiology of ageing by applying common sense and everyday observations. In general terms, as we age we gradually wear out. This is true of all the bodily systems but is more apparent in some than others. As a rule of thumb, from the age of 50 we lose about 1% per year of the functioning cells of our kidneys. This does not result in a difference in effectiveness that can be detected by routine tests or patient symptoms, because the human body is equipped with an inbuilt reserve, with capacity to tolerate large demands or stresses before it begins to fail. Serum creatinine is a breakdown product of muscle creatine phosphate and is produced by the body at a constant rate and filtered out of the blood by the kidneys. Measuring serum creatinine is simple to do and is a universally accepted measure of kidney function. However, this has some limitations, not least because the rate of production of creatinine is dependent on muscle mass. As muscle mass normally diminishes with age, any concomitant deterioration in renal function may be masked, and will not necessarily be reflected by a rise in serum creatinine.

At the same time that physiological decline occurs there is an increased risk of developing significant degenerative disease. This will include conditions which have implications with respect to the kidneys, such as hypertension, diabetes and atherosclerotic disease. Not only do these conditions all have the potential to accentuate the natural decline in renal function, but the drugs used to treat them frequently have toxic effects on the kidneys. The combination of physiological ageing, accumulation of chronic conditions and the increasing burden of medications reduces the ability of older peoples' kidneys to deal with additional stresses. It also increases their susceptibility to acute injury.

Terminology

The term acute kidney injury (AKI) has largely replaced the term acute renal failure (ARF). The change in terminology is intended to reflect the spectrum of injury that can occur with this condition and the importance of a targeted response. At the less severe end of the spectrum effective treatment may consist of increasing a patient's oral fluid intake and adjusting their medication, whereas at the other extreme dialysis and management by the specialist team may be required. Clinically, AKI is characterised by a sudden deterioration in kidney function resulting in the body's inability to moderate fluid balance, electrolyte and metabolic homeostasis. **Although AKI is frequently reversible, prompt identification and appropriate treatment is important to reduce the risks of permanent kidney damage or death**.

Acute kidney injury is increasingly common, particularly in hospitalised patients. It is associated with high levels of morbidity and mortality, with only 50% of patients surviving to six months, of whom a significant proportion remain dialysis-dependent. Although the actual incidence in the UK is unknown, an incidence of around 486 per million population has been estimated. The incidence in older people is higher because of pre-existing renal impairment and co-existing conditions, particularly vascular diseases such as diabetes and cardiac disease. Arteriosclerosis in renal blood vessels is increasingly common with advancing age, even in the absence of other comorbidities. Vascular changes lead to scarring and fibrosis of kidney tissue, which is accelerated in the presence of more generalised atherosclerosis and hypertension and leads to kidney injury. Patients with sepsis, hypotension or hypovolaemia are also at an increased risk of AKI, as are those taking medications such as non-steroidal anti-inflammatory drugs (NSAIDs), diuretics and angiotensin converting enzyme inhibitors (ACE inhibitors).

AKI is a serious condition and has an associated mortality ranging between 10% and 80%. In hospitalised patients it may occur through a pre-existing or presenting condition or subsequent iatrogenic injury following admission.Patients with AKI are typically admitted for reasons other than a kidney problem and tend to be managed initially in non-specialist areas, usually by comparatively junior doctors. For this reason it is important that all those responsible for patient care can identify those at risk of AKI and initiate an appropriate response. This may include preventative measures such as rehydration, preliminary investigations, commencing treatment and referral to a more senior colleague or specialist service such as radiology or the kidney team.

Definition of acute kidney injury

AKI is characterised by a rapid fall in glomerular filtration rate (GFR) and an abrupt and sustained rise in urea, electrolytes and creatinine. It can induce life-threatening fluid and electrolyte imbalances. The recent Renal Association guidelines consider the presence of **one** of the following scenarios as initial confirmation of AKI:

Table 6.1 The main causes of AKI.

Pre-renal	Intra-renal	Intra-renal	Intra-renal	Intra-renal	Post-renal
Reduced blood flow	**Affecting glomeruli**	**Affecting tubules**	**Affecting interstitium**	**Affecting blood vessels**	**Urinary tract obstruction**
Hypotension Anaphylactic or cardiogenic shock	**Inflammatory** Glomerulonephritis	**Ischaemic** Prolonged renal hypoperfusion	**Drug-induced** NSAIDs, antibiotics	**Vasculitis** e.g. Wegener's	**Intrinsic** Bladder tumours, stones
Hypovolaemia Diarrhoea and vomiting, haemorrhage	**Thrombotic** Accelerated hypertension, haemolytic uraemic syndrome	**Toxic** NSAIDs, radiocontrast	**Granulomatous** sarcoidosis	**Cholesterol emboli**	**Extrinsic** Enlarged prostate, pelvic tumours
Renal artery disease Stenosis, occlusion		**Metabolic** Hypercalcaemia	**Infiltrative** Lymphoma		

- a rise in serum creatinine ≥26 μmol/L within 48 hours
- a rise in serum creatinine ≥1.5-fold from the reference value, which is known or presumed to have occurred within one week
- reduced urine output <0.5 mL/kg/h for more than six consecutive hours

A reference value may be available from the patient's general practitioner and may indicate whether the rise in serum creatinine is acute or long-standing. If not available, the serum creatinine should be repeated within 24 hours.

Aetiology and outcome

The causes of AKI can be categorised into pre-renal, intra-renal (intrinsic) and post-renal causes (Table 6.1). Pre-renal causes of AKI are most commonly factors such as hypotension and hypovolaemia which cause reduced blood flow to the kidney. In patients with pre-renal AKI, prompt intervention to rehydrate and improve the patient's blood pressure will often prevent the progression to established kidney damage, namely acute tubular necrosis (ATN). Intra-renal causes of AKI result in direct injury to the renal tissue and may involve the kidney blood vessels, tubules, interstitium or glomeruli.

The most common causes of AKI in hospitals are pre-renal: under-perfusion of the kidneys, usually due to hypovolaemia and/or relative hypotension (Table 6.2). Elderly patients are at particular risk because of the problems associated with maintaining adequate hydration in hospital and the increased likelihood of an inelastic vasculature. If left untreated, under-perfusion is likely to lead to ATN, which can last days or weeks and may result in permanent damage to the kidneys.

Approach to the patient

Many of these patients can present very unwell, and while this seems obvious it is still worth mentioning that recognising acutely unwell patients is the key to timely interventions. The generic 'ABC' approach to achieve some stability is always the first priority. Assuming the patient is stable and in a safe clinical environment, then the general principles of taking a history, examination, investigations and management can be implemented (Table 6.3). The initial aim is to determine whether the kidney dysfunction is due to a pre-renal, intra-renal or post-renal cause.

Physical examination

The most crucial part of the physical examination (Table 6.4) in the initial stages of management is to ensure there is no urinary retention and to correctly assess the fluid balance of the patient. While patients may present with

Table 6.2 The commonest causes of hospital-acquired AKI.

45% of cases	Acute tubular necrosis	Secondary to acute tubular damage, often multifactorial including sepsis, hypotension and use of nephrotoxic drugs
25%	Acute tubular necrosis (postoperative)	Mostly due to pre-renal causes
12%	Acute contrast nephropathy	

In intensive care the most common cause is sepsis, usually in association with multi-organ failure

Table 6.3 Clinical history.

Pre-existing conditions	Hypertension, diabetes, cardiac disease, vascular disease, chronic kidney disease. Conditions affecting urinary outflow, e.g. enlarged prostate, pelvic tumour or previous stones
Recent acute illness	Associated with excess fluid loss, e.g. fever, diarrhoea and vomiting or reduced fluid intake
New medications	In particular ACE inhibitors, ARBs, antibiotics and NSAIDs. Also check over-the-counter medications and herbal remedies (see Chapter 8)
Symptoms that suggest systemic disease	Rashes, joint pains, myalgia, acute deafness, recurrent sinusitis or haemoptysis
Symptoms of advanced chronic kidney disease	Nausea, vomiting, weight loss, fatigue, itching, nocturia or hiccups
Family history of kidney disease	Polycystic kidneys, Alport syndrome

fluid retention and oedema, many are dehydrated. It is not always possible to detect a large bladder on abdominal examination, and some form of ultrasonic imaging is mandatory. Urinary retention in females is unusual, and if it occurs careful examination of lower limb neurology is necessary to exclude spinal cord pathology.

In older people the commonly used signs to gauge fluid depletion can be misleading. An elevated jugular venous pressure, basal crackles and oedema can usually be safely interpreted as showing excess fluid, but it is often more difficult to determine whether the patient is dry. It is important to note here that intensely ill patients can have gross oedema at the same time as being intravascularly dehydrated. Poor skin turgor and dry mouth become an increasingly common finding in healthy older people and cannot be relied upon to indicate dehydration. More useful signs include postural hypotension, which, in the acutely unwell,

Table 6.4 Physical examination.

Volume status	Pulse rate, blood pressure, jugular venous pressure, dry mouth, reduced skin turgor, pulmonary crepitations (auscultation), peripheral oedema (extent of)
Systemic disease	Fever, splinter haemorrhages, skin rashes, joint swelling/tenderness, iritis or scleritis, new heart murmurs
Vascular disease	Cool peripheries, absent peripheral pulses, abdominal aortic aneurysm (palpable), vascular bruits
Advanced chronic kidney disease	Pallor, uraemic discoloration (yellow tinge) of the skin, excoriations, pericardial rub
Hypertension: long-standing or severe	Retinopathy, e.g. haemorrhages, papilloedema
Bladder outflow obstruction	Palpable bladder, abdominal pain

is most commonly due to intravascular volume depletion. Measurement of blood pressure while the patient is supine may be falsely reassuring. If the patient is well enough to stand or even to sit upright the blood pressure in this position should also be recorded. A significant drop in postural blood pressure (>20 mmHg in systolic pressure) may be taken as indicating significant intravascular volume depletion. Other good indicators of volume depletion include a low jugular venous pressure and a lack of axillary moisture. In a hospital environment some sweat production is normal, so if a patient's armpit is bone-dry this is a good indicator that he or she is dehydrated. So while it is not the most pleasant place to explore, checking a patient's armpit can be very informative. A number of tests should be performed on all patients suspected of AKI (Table 6.5), as well as urinalysis, which can indicate a number of conditions (Table 6.6).

Acute or chronic kidney disease?

Establishing whether the patient has acute or chronic kidney disease is impor-tant, because the management will differ. Patients with chronic kidney disease (CKD) whose kidney function has worsened progressively over time (as opposed to acutely) may present with stage 5 CKD, in which any recovery of kidney function is unlikely. These patients should be referred to the specialist team for assessment and long-term management.

Previous creatinine levels

Previous creatinine levels (if available) are the most useful in determining whether or not the patient had pre-existing renal impairment. If there are a

Table 6.5 Investigations: the following tests should be performed on all patients in whom AKI is suspected.

Full blood count	A raised white cell count may indicate an infective aetiology. Normochromic normocytic anaemia may indicate a chronic renal problem.
Urea and electrolytes (U&Es)	Essential for the diagnosis. Look out for rising potassium, as the treatment of this can be an emergency. Also helpful to look for previous creatinine levels to indicate whether this is acute, chronic or an acute deterioration on a background of chronic renal impairment (acute-on-chronic renal failure).
Glucose	New-onset diabetes can present with extreme dehydration, acidosis and renal failure.
C-reactive protein	This is a good indicator of an ongoing inflammatory or infective process. Can also be used to monitor response to therapy.
Calcium	High calcium levels can cause an osmotic diuresis and subsequent dehydration and renal failure, but lower levels may point to a more chronic renal problem – often associated with a high serum phosphate.
Blood gases	These are particularly useful in determining the acid–base balance and can indicate the extent of any acidosis, which may be life threatening.
Chest x-ray	Looking for signs of fluid overload or infection.
Renal tract ultrasound	This will reliably determine whether there is any obstruction to the renal system. This is essential and should be done as an emergency, as any obstruction will require immediate treatment.
Antibodies	Assays for autoimmune diseases which can affect the kidneys should be requested when there are signs or symptoms of systemic disease. ANCA, ANA, anti-glomerular basement membrane (GBM) antibody can usually be done urgently but need liaison with your local immunology laboratory.
Urine	The urine should be collected and tested on the ward with a routine dipstick analysis. This will give an indication of the presence of protein, blood, leucocytes and nitrites. Positive nitrites and leucocytes would support a diagnosis of infection. Blood and protein can be helpful when considering causes of intra-renal kidney disease.

Table 6.6 Urinalysis.

Urine dipstick	Reduced renal blood flow	Glomerular disease	Tubular damage	Interstitial disease	Urinary tract obstruction
Blood	Negative	Strongly positive (2+ to 4+)	Negative	May be positive (trace to 1+)	Usually negative (unless co-existent infection)
Protein	Negative	Strongly positive (2+ to 4+)	May be positive (trace to 2+)	May be positive (trace to 2+)	Usually negative (unless co-existent infection)

number of previous measurements taken over time it is also possible to estimate the degree of impairment and the rate of any decline. There is some controversy in the literature whether estimated GFR (eGFR) provides more clinical information regarding AKI than changes in serum creatinine (see Chapter 3).

Ultrasound

In patients with CKD an ultrasound will often show smaller than normal kidneys with a reduced cortical thickness.

Signs and symptoms of kidney disease

Patients with CKD are likely to have anaemia, with high phosphate and low calcium levels, and while patients with AKI may have similarly deranged laboratory results this is much less common. Patients with advanced CKD (stage 4/5) will often report long duration and insidious onset of symptoms such as fatigue, nocturia, nausea or itch (but note that these are also common in elderly patients without kidney problems). Patients with AKI typically present with an acute illness such as pneumonia, diarrhoea or sepsis.

Urinary obstruction

In situations where the cause of AKI is not apparent, patients should be asked about any problems associated with the renal tract including kidney stones or bladder outflow obstruction, typical symptoms being urinary hesitancy, frequency and nocturia. Feel for an enlarged bladder but remember that in people with chronic retention the bladder can become atonic and often difficult to appreciate on abdominal examination. Complete lack of urine output (anuria) is rare and should always raise the suspicion of obstruction. This can be excluded with imaging - usually ultrasound.

Urinalysis

Urine should be tested using a dipstick and sent for microscopy. The presence of blood and protein on dipstick raises the possibility of glomerular disease or vasculitis, and the patient should be referred to a nephrologist.

Other investigations

These may include (usually under the direction of a nephrologist):

- Bence Jones protein and serum protein electrophoresis (multiple myeloma)
- kidney biopsy – usually indicated by a lack of recovery, and managed in specialist services

Management and prevention

Where to manage patients with AKI?

It is not necessary or feasible for all patients with AKI to be transferred to specialist kidney services. With the right monitoring and medical management, most patients with AKI can be safely managed in non-specialist areas. This is particularly so in the case of many elderly patients, who may be more appropriately managed in older people services with input from the multidisciplinary team. In many instances, patients with complex chronic problems and a poor prognosis will be clinically unsuitable for dialysis. This should be considered before referral or transfer to specialist services. The prognosis of frail and elderly patients with AKI is contingent not just upon restoring kidney function, but upon preserving and promoting global functional independence. In most instances, this is more likely to be achieved in an elderly care setting with regular input from other disciplines such as occupational and physiotherapy.

As AKI is frequently preventable, it is important to identify those patients at risk and initiate preventative measures (Box 6.1).

Phases of AKI

The management of AKI can be broadly divided into three phases (Table 6.7). The **initial phase** represents a period during which, if identified and treated promptly (for instance with appropriate fluid resuscitation), any damage to the kidney is potentially reversible. If the patient remains oliguric despite rehydration and an adequate blood pressure, they are likely to have progressed to the maintenance phase. The **maintenance phase** indicates that acute tubular necrosis is likely to have occurred and, although still recoverable, this may continue for several weeks. During this phase, patients are often fluid restricted to reduce the risk of fluid overload. The **recovery phase** may be characterised by a polyuric phase in which patients may pass several litres of fluid a day and will require careful monitoring.

Box 6.1   Identifying high-risk patients and prevention

The key to prevention is early identification of those patients at risk, including elderly patients and those with any of the following:

- diabetes
- hypertension
- vascular disease
- pre-existing kidney disease

For those patients at risk, preventative measures include:

- maintaining an adequate circulating volume and blood pressure
- avoidance of nephrotoxic medications and contrast mediums

Triggers for reassessing hydration status of susceptible patients:

- prolonged fasting: because of unforeseen delays in theatre lists etc., patients may be fasted for longer than intended
- pyrexial illness: fluid loss during pyrexial illness may be underestimated
- hot weather
- physical inability of patient to drink/tolerate replacement volumes required
- confused patients
- lack of facilities for patients to help themselves to drinks, or patient requires help to drink
- over-effective diuretics

Table 6.7   Phases of AKI (after Pratt & Nouri 2009).

Initial phase	Time from initial insult to reduction in kidney function. Renal damage is potentially reversible.
Maintenance phase	Established kidney damage. Phase lasts days to weeks Recovery may be sporadic and non-linear.
Recovery phase	Urea and creatinine levels returning towards pre-injury levels. Usually a polyuric phase which requires careful management.

In patients who have AKI, early senior medical input is essential. Depending on the severity and response to initial treatment, there may need to be consultation with specialist renal services. AKI is a medical emergency, and those patients requiring renal replacement therapy will need to be managed in critical care or renal high dependency units (for more details on this visit the Renal Association website).

> ## Box 6.2 Management of medical emergencies in AKI
>
> **Electrolyte imbalances** – Consider bicarbonate infusion for extreme acidosis. For hyperkalaemia consider bolus or infusion of dextrose 50% via a large blood vessel (with insulin if the patient is diabetic). Salbutamol nebulisers may be administered alone or in conjunction with dextrose (see Chapter 8). Replace other depleted electrolytes such as calcium, magnesium. Consider monitoring using a cardiac monitor.
>
> **Pulmonary oedema** – Prescribe oxygen (hospitals increasingly have a group directive for oxygen administration) and monitor saturations, respiratory effort and pattern. Consider sedation and intubation if delay in filtration/dialysisis anticipated. Diuretics may not be effective, particularly in standard doses. A challenge of high-dose diuretics may be tried under specialist advice.

The management of AKI includes treating the particular cause of AKI, but also involves more general measures associated with managing ATN, which is the commonest case of AKI:

● Full set of observations, including assessment for shock and hypovolaemia.
● Identification and treatment of hyperkalamia, acidosis and pulmonary oedema. Individually, each of these constitutes a medical emergency. Immediate initiation of treatment should be considered even in patients awaiting transfer to specialist services (Box 6.2).
● Identification and management of treatable causes. Correct hypovolaemia with appropriate fluids and aim to restore an appropriate blood pressure. This may require 250 mL boluses of gelofusine until volume replete. Insert a urinary catheter. If there is an obstruction at the bladder outflow level then this may be difficult and you may need to consult a urologist to consider a suprapubic approach. Sometimes the obstruction is at a higher level than the bladder and a nephrostomy tube may need to be inserted directly into the kidney (refer to a radiologist). These patients are usually managed in a specialist centre and require immediate intervention to reduce the risk of dialysis dependency.
● Review medications. Stop all potentially nephrotoxic drugs, particularly NSAIDs, ACE inhibitors or angiotensin receptor blockers (ARBs), metformin and potassium-sparing diuretics. Adjust doses of renally excreted medications (see current *British National Formulary* or *Handbook of Renal Medicine*). Stop diuretics and antihypertensives if appropriate (for instance if the patient is dehydrated or there is relative hypotension).
● Monitor and regulate fluid input and record hourly fluid output. Set a fluid target each day, noting that insensible losses account for approximately 500 mL every 24 hours. Observations should be made at least four-hourly. Arrange to have the patient weighed daily, preferably first thing in the morning.

- Optimal nutrition requires a high-calorie diet, and the patient's urea and electrolytes may require a restriction in foods high in protein and/or potassium. The extent of any dietary restriction needs to be tempered against the patient's appetite and food intake, as most severely ill patients are anorexic (see Chapter 9). Referral to a renal dietitian is recommended.
- Identification and treatment of any infection. Indwelling lines and catheters should be checked at regular intervals and removed at the earliest opportunity.
- Identification and treatment of any bleeding tendency. Avoid aspirin and start a proton-pump inhibitor (PPI) in high-risk patients (note the association of PPIs with the increased risk of *Clostridium difficile*-associated disease).

Referral to the renal specialists

All patients with suspicion of renal inflammatory disease (blood and protein on urine dipstick) should be referred. Other patients should be referred either to renal services or to critical care if there is hyperkalaemia, pulmonary oedema, acidosis, pericarditis or uraemic encephalopathy. Patients will require review by a nephrologist for suitability for longer-term dialysis or follow-up for persistent chronic renal impairment if recovery from the acute illness is incomplete.

Medical emergencies

Electrolyte imbalances and pulmonary oedema constitute medical emergencies and require an urgent nephrology review. In the first instance, this may involve a telephone discussion to ensure the appropriate treatment is initiated to stabilise the patient before transfer. This is particularly important if the specialist centre is based in another hospital. Try to avoid transferring patients during the night.

AKI and heart failure

A significant proportion of patients with AKI have other vascular conditions which can complicate their management and restrict treatment options. In addition, AKI can precipitate a number of cardiac conditions such as arrhythmias, myocardial infarction, cardiac arrest and congestive heart failure. Up to 35% of patients with AKI experience cardiovascular complications. In patients with pre-existing heart failure, the use of ACE inhibitors, ARBs and large doses of diuretics can accentuate the risk of AKI and lead to therapeutic dilemmas, particularly when cardiac function is poor. In these circumstances careful consideration must be given to the patient's overall condition and prognosis. In some instances the optimal treatment regime will be palliative. In others the trade-off is optimising cardiac output at the cost of worsening kidney function. Treatment options are often complicated by chronic hypotension and large amounts of extracellular fluid. Although dialysis may be considered as a treatment option for patients with heart failure and AKI, it is technically difficult to effectively dialyse chronically hypotensive patients, and specialist advice should be sought early in these circumstances. In these situations it is important that patient and carer expectations are not raised inappropriately, as only a small number of these patients are likely to be considered clinically suitable for dialysis.

Prognosis

Providing an accurate estimate of an individual's chances of recovery is always a challenge to any healthcare professional. We are often surprised by patients' capacity to recover despite seemingly irreversible catastrophic pathology. With this in mind, however, an episode of AKI is a serious event, and even if the injury to the kidneys is reversible, the consequent stresses on other organs is more profound. Despite advances in medical technology and management regimes, the total mortality associated with AKI has remained unchanged for several decades, with only 50% of patients surviving to six months. The prognosis is likely to be worse in older people. A high proportion of deaths associated with AKI occur during the patient's initial admission. However uncertain the prognosis, it is good practice to discuss this with the patient and family at regular intervals, even if this is limited to explaining the uncertainties and a range of possible scenarios.

Generally, older patients experience a higher rate of complications and have poorer outcomes in the initial stages of AKI management than younger patients. The longer-term prognosis will depend on the underlying conditions and frailty of the individual.

It may be helpful to think of patients as belonging to three main groups, those with poor, good and uncertain prognosis.

Poor prognosis

These are the patients in whom the chances of recovery from the current illness is vanishingly small. Even very experienced physicians can have difficulty in reliably recognising patients who will not survive. The following clinical signs may indicate patients who are unlikely to survive the acute illness:

- several organs showing signs of failure
- previously poor function (e.g. being bed-bound)
- low blood pressure despite fluid resuscitation
- drowsiness and confusion
- pressure ulcers
- persistent oliguria in spite of fluid therapy

For those who continue to have a grave prognosis in spite of optimal treatment, the immediate issues are how best to communicate the prognosis to the patient and his/her loved ones, and when to change focus from active treatment to a more palliative approach. There is no easy way to deal with either of these issues, but bearing the following principles in mind may help:

(1) Try to be honest. Patients who are very unwell are often delirious or drowsy (or both), and may be unable to have anything but a superficial conversation about their situation. Those who are lucid and able to discuss their future should be offered the opportunity to talk about their treatment and care. Many people welcome the opportunity to do this but are hesitant about raising the issues themselves. It can be particularly helpful to determine the patient's own views about how aggressive treatment should be, and where this should be delivered – many people would prefer to be at home (with support) rather than in hospital if the treatments being given are unlikely to be successful.

(2) For confused patients, try to determine what the person's views were before they were ill. With the rising awareness of advance directives, these are becoming more common, and must be respected when considering treatment of 'incapable' adults. There are important differences between advance directives and advance care plans which practitioners should be aware of (see NHS Choices). Even if there is no formal record of the patient's wishes, the family may be able to give an outline of what they believe the patient would want. This can be helpful when deciding on treatment strategies.

(3) Be sure to speak to loved ones (with the patient's consent where appropriate) to make sure they realise the gravity of the situation. Many complaints from families or loved ones stem from a misunderstanding of the severity of illness, and this can be avoided by taking the time to talk at an early stage, and subsequently at regular intervals, even when there is little new to convey.

(4) Remember that it is the medical staff who make the decisions about medical care. It is good practice to consult with families and carers etc., but it is not appropriate to put the decision making into their hands. This potentially places a burden on them and can lead to feelings of guilt, uncertainty and anxiety. These decisions can be very difficult, but that is what healthcare professionals are trained and paid to do.

(5) Make clear plans in the patient record which all staff (and, where appropriate, family) are aware of. This should include the ceiling level of care that should be offered if the patient's condition deteriorates. For instance, ventilation may not be appropriate in patients with long-standing respiratory conditions.

(6) Decide on the appropriateness of attempting resuscitation if the patient were to die. For most hospitals there is a default position of resuscitation attempts unless a decision is made to the contrary. It is important to avoid the situation of subjecting a dying patient to such assaults simply because the decision has not been considered.

(7) If you do not think a treatment is going to help, then consider carefully why it is being given. This sounds like common sense, but it is surprising how many very old and frail people die whilst receiving treatments which in retrospect were never going to be helpful in the short term. Consider stopping drugs which may be causing side effects. They can always be restarted at a later stage if the situation changes.

(8) If the patient recovers from this illness, take the opportunity to talk about their wishes for future care if they were to suffer another serious illness. If the patient does wish to refuse aspects of care then encourage him or her to register a formal advance directive with the general practitioner after discharge. Making a will and appointing a lasting power of attorney are also to be encouraged.

(9) If it appears that the patient is in the final stages of his or her life, consider starting an end-of-life pathway. Most acute hospitals use a care template such as the Liverpool Care Pathway, and there is one specifically for use in patients with kidney impairment. These pathways help to ensure that the appropriate strategies are used to keep a patient comfortable whilst avoiding unnecessary or unpleasant interventions.

(10) Similarly, in circumstances where patients are still receiving active treatment but the outlook remains poor, consider using an end-of-life pathway and recording the treatment intervention as a variance. The difficulty in diagnosing dying should not be a barrier to pre-empting and preparing for the possibility that the patient may not survive.

Good prognosis

A good prognosis may be considered when:

(1) there appears to be a single precipitating factor causing the renal dysfunction, such as dehydration or urinary outflow obstruction
(2) the patient was previously well and independent with everyday activities
(3) there is prompt improvement with initial therapy
(4) the patient maintains a good blood pressure
(5) the patient remains lucid with no confusion

The prompt identification and treatment of the cause of AKI may lead to a rapid improvement in the patient's condition and biochemistry. Even in patients in whom a good recovery is expected, it should always be borne in mind that complications frequently occur in elderly patients. The common problems encountered are confusion (delirium), functional decline (manifested as difficulty in performing everyday tasks such as getting out of bed, walking, getting dressed), falls, infections, pressure ulcers and incontinence. When these complications occur it can lead to a progressive spiral of decline which is difficult to explain or reverse. The trick is to try to avoid the complications happening rather than deal with them after they have occurred. This is best achieved by having an awareness of the potential issues from all of the multidisciplinary team who are caring for the patient. The principles are:

(1) Keep the patient mobile:
    (a) encourage the patient to walk to the toilet and around the ward
    (b) get the patient's walking aid if one is used at home
    (c) ensure the patient has the correct footwear
(2) Avoid drugs which will make things worse:
    (a) such as sedatives
    (b) be aware of withdrawal from drugs, including alcohol
(3) Pay attention to the environment:
    (a) avoid excessive noise
    (b) give visual cues to where the patient is (e.g. hospital signage)
    (c) allow access to toileting facilities
(4) Involve all the team nurses, physiotherapists, occupational therapists etc., and the patient's family.
(5) Optimise sensory input – clocks, hearing aids, prompts.
(6) Avoid unnecessary moves either within or between wards.
(7) Control symptoms such as pain and constipation.
(8) Be aware that there may be more than one pathology, and manage accordingly.

The importance of ongoing monitoring

The multidisciplinary team plays an important role in the ongoing monitoring of the patient's condition. Where possible the same small group of nurses should be used, to optimise continuity of care. Important changes can be subtle. Encourage the family to be involved and ask at regular intervals how they think the patient is doing. Recognising these changes and reporting accordingly can pre-empt rapid deterioration. As well as the usual monitoring associated with hospital inpatients, such as an early warning score, it is useful to think more qualitatively when assessing the patient's condition (Box 6.3).

Acute care is increasingly populated by older, and often sicker, patients. Therefore everybody practising in the acute sector should be developing their skills in looking after older people. It is good practice to discuss with patients their views on treatment and escalation of care as above, even when they are considered to have a good prognosis.

Uncertain prognosis

This will probably be the most common situation encountered. In the acute setting the prognosis will become more apparent depending on how the patient responds to initial treatments. During this phase of management it is important to devise a contingency plan should the patient not improve with first-line treatments. The main dilemma is usually whether the patient is likely to benefit from escalation of care to high dependency or specialist renal services.

> ## Box 6.3 Ongoing monitoring
>
> - Daily weight is often a more accurate indicator of fluid balance than an intake and output chart. Observe for cumulative weight gain or loss over several days (1 kg equivalent to 1 litre of fluid). Assess the extent of any oedema and whether it is increasing (in bed-bound patients check for increasing sacral oedema).
> - Observe respiratory pattern and use of accessory muscles. Is the patient having difficulty speaking because of breathlessness? Fluid retention is not always evenly distributed, and patients can have pulmonary oedema with little or no peripheral oedema.
> - Patients who are fluid restricted may need support to keep within fluid allowance. Note the 'hidden' fluid content of certain foods (see Chapter 9). Don't tempt patients who are fluid restricted with a full water jug.
> - Identify related signs on which to base action, and develop an anticipatory plan. So, for instance, what to do when a patient is considered euvolaemic but is still not passing urine, or if blood pressure remains low despite adequate rehydration. Pre-emptively consider criteria for escalation to high dependency, for instance if inotropes are indicated.
> - Observe for changes in functional status. Recovery is often non-linear, but is the patient regaining the strength to be able to do more for him- or herself? Relatives and healthcare assistants are often sensitive to subtle changes in a patient's functional ability.

When to escalate care

If a patient is responding to the initial treatments given on arrival, then it is reasonable to continue that approach. If, however the response is not good, then very quickly complications will arise. The main indicators that things are not going well are:

- worsening acidosis
- patient is becoming fluid overloaded and not passing adequate urine
- high and/or rising potassium levels
- the failure of other organs

When these sort of events start happening then a decision needs to be taken about what to do next. It is very difficult to actively manage these problems outside of a critical care area, as they may require invasive monitoring and renal replacement therapy (RRT).

The question then arises of who should be moved to the intensive care unit for invasive treatment or transfer to specialist services, which may be situated at another hospital, and when should we accept that the deterioration heralds the end stages of that person's life, in which case a palliative approach would be more appropriate. These decisions are best taken by a senior clinician involved with the patient's care, informed by knowledge of the person's previous level of function, and expressed wishes if known, and with an idea of how reversible the underlying pathology is.

At one extreme, if a person has previously been very dependent for all aspects of daily living, has more than one chronic disease, and presents with AKI in the context of sepsis-induced multi-organ failure, then the chances of recovery would be small even with very intensive treatment. In these circumstances many clinicians would tend towards taking a conservative approach with a defined ceiling of care at the ward level. At the other end of the spectrum it would be reasonable to consider a higher level of care, even for a very old person, if that person had previously been independent with good exercise tolerance and had acute kidney injury, for instance, secondary to dehydration from a bout of viral diarrhoea (which one would expect to resolve relatively quickly).

Box 6.4   Case study: an older patient with pre-existing kidney impairment

An 87-year-old man was admitted to an acute medical ward during an episode of diarrhoea that had started seven days previously following a trip to India. He had a history of a cerebrovascular injury that had left him bed-bound and heavily dependent on his family, with whom he lived. He had also had two previous myocardial infarctions, as well as atrial fibrillation, heart failure, type 2 diabetes and hypertension. On admission he was unresponsive, severely dehydrated, with a systolic blood pressure of 70 mmHg. Blood tests indicated a creatinine of 435 mmol/L, with very low levels of magnesium and calcium. The patient's records indicated a baseline creatinine in the previous year of 187 mmol/L, indicating pre-existing renal impairment.

The management plan was to rehydrate and correct the electrolyte imbalance. Given the patient's medical history and frail state the decision was made not to escalate care should he deteriorate further, and a do not resuscitate order was filed. Fluid and electrolyte replacement began with several boluses of a plasma expander followed by several litres of various solutions. Over several hours the patient's urine output increased to around 50 mL per hour and his systolic blood pressure reached 95 mmHg. He was more lucid and was able to communicate with his family. Further blood tests over several days indicated an improvement in the patient's urea and electrolytes. Although his creatinine did not return to its baseline level, once the patient felt well enough, early discharge was possible because of his family's long-term care arrangements and the agreement of his GP to monitor his condition. The patient was referred to the renal palliative care team for supportive care.

These decisions are often difficult ones to make. The ethical considerations can be complex, and the science inexact. It is helpful to take the decision in consultation with all interested parties, including the ICU and/or the renal specialist, and to be prepared to reconsider if events or circumstances change (Box 6.4).

As a general rule, it is recommended that a person's quality of life should be kept out of the decision-making process unless the patient has expressed a view. It is not possible to estimate someone else's quality of life, and assumptions based on subjective opinion of what sort of life would be worth living can be very misleading.

Advance care plans and advance decisions to refuse treatments

Advance care plans and decisions to refuse treatments include the concept of ensuring agreement between a patient and his or her healthcare providers about what treatment plans should be instituted for that patient. When these have been drawn up by a patient correctly they need to be respected. For further information and guidance on their use and application please refer to current guidance which is published on the National End of Life Care Programme website.

Lasting power of attorney

Lasting power of attorney (LPA) is a term that was introduced in the Mental Capacity Act (2005). It provides a new role which is more extensive than the old enduring power of attorney (EPA). An EPA enabled a person to nominate someone else to act on his or her behalf in the event of an illness which led to the loss of mental capacity. The EPA, however, only gave the nominated party the right to handle financial affairs. The powers of an LPA have been extended to potentially include decisions relating to health care. A person can decide when drawing up an LPA agreement whether it should include just financial matters or also include health and welfare decisions – and if this is so, then that person must be involved in significant decisions about the patient's treatment.

Conclusion

Many hospitalised patients are at risk of developing acute kidney injury, but older people are particularly so. Whilst the management of AKI is principally the same irrespective of age, older people are more likely to have pre-existing chronic conditions and/or frailty, which can complicate and constrain management options. Primarily managing the person and not the disease will help to ensure that treatment decisions are made in the context of the patient's capacity to benefit and their wishes regarding their current and future care.

References and resources

Ashley, C. & Currie A. (2009). *The Renal Drug Handbook*, 3rd edition. Radcliffe Medical Press, Oxford.

BNF (2012) *British National Formulary 63*. British Medical Association and Royal Pharmaceutical Society of Great Britain, London.

Brincat, S. & Hilton, R. (2008) Prevention of acute kidney injury. *British Journal of HospitalMedicine*, **69**, 450–4.

Edinburgh Royal Infirmary Renal Unit (Edren). General information regarding kidney disease and treatments for professionals, patients and the public. They also have a sister website where they have published an electronic website and various patient pathways. http://www.edren.org and http://www.edrep.org (accessed September 2012).

Lewington, A. & Kanagasundaram, S. (2011) Renal Association acute kidney injury guidelines. http://www.renal.org/clinical/GuidelinesSection/AcuteKidneyInjury.aspx (accessed September 2012).

Liverpool Care Pathway for the Dying Patient (LCP). http://www.mcpcil.org.uk (accessed September 2012).

Mental Capacity Act (2005) http://www.legislation.gov.uk/ukpga/2005/9 (accessed September 2012).

NHS Choices. Consent to treatment. http://www.nhs.uk/conditions/consent-to-treatment/Pages/Introduction.aspx (accessed September 2012).

NHS End of Life Care Programme. http://www.endoflifecareforadults.nhs.uk (accessed September 2012).

Pratt, M. & Nouri, P. (2009) Acute renal failure. In: *Handbook of Nephrology and Hypertension*, 6th edition (ed. C. S. Wilcox & C. C. Tisher), pp. 277–89. Wolters Kluwer/Lippincott Williams & Wilkins, Philadelphia.

Renal Association. The professional organisation for nephrologists (including trainees) and scientists in the UK. http://www.renal.org (accessed September 2012).

Workeneh, B.T., Agraharkar, M. & Gupta, R. (2012) Acute renal failure. *Medscape Reference*. http://emedicine.medscape.com/article/243492 (accessed September 2012).

Chapter 7

Management of Patients with or at Risk of Kidney Disease on the Surgical Ward

Colin H. Jones and Maggie Higginbotham

York Teaching Hospital NHS Foundation Trust, York, UK

Introduction

The kidneys are very vulnerable to injury in patients admitted to hospital for other reasons. New-onset kidney injury can occur in people with previously normal kidney function (acute kidney injury). Kidney function can worsen further in those with existing kidney disease (acute-on-chronic kidney injury). Care must be taken with prescribed medications which can either induce or contribute to kidney injury or, if excreted by the kidneys, may accumulate leading to toxicity. Standard management protocols in the pre-, peri- and postoperative period may need modifying, both to prevent deterioration in kidney function and to avoid predictable complications in those with existing kidney failure.

Patient population

The spectrum of kidney disease includes:

- Acute kidney injury (AKI) – Baseline kidney function is normal; kidney function deteriorates quickly; there is potential for recovery of normal kidney function.
- Acute-on-chronic kidney disease – Baseline kidney function is abnormal; kidney function deteriorates further from baseline over a short time period;

Kidney Disease Management: A Practical Approach for the Non-Specialist Healthcare Practitioner, First Edition. Edited by Rachel Lewis and Helen Noble.
© 2013 John Wiley & Sons, Ltd. Published 2013 by John Wiley & Sons, Ltd.

there is potential for recovery of kidney function to baseline, but not to normal kidney function.

- Chronic kidney disease (CKD) – Baseline kidney function is abnormal; kidney function has deteriorated slowly; there is no potential for recovery of kidney function.
- Stage 5 CKD
  - Dialysis – the patient is on regular dialysis treatment.
  - Transplant – the patient has a functioning kidney transplant.

While stage 5 CKD is quite rare (100 per million population in UK), CKD is common (5% of the population have stage 1/2 and a further 5% stage 3/4 CKD: Stevens *et al.* 2007). CKD is a major risk factor for developing acute-on-chronic kidney injury as a hospital inpatient.

Recognising kidney injury

The priority is to identify high-risk patients and to *avoid* kidney injury in hospital inpatients. However, if kidney injury does occur it is important to recognise it as early as possible. Many patients will be identified using early warning or acute illness scores, which will include pulse rate, blood pressure, respiratory rate.

More specific markers of worsening kidney injury include:

- **Serum creatinine** – If the serum creatinine is rising by more than 50-100 µmol/L/day, then the patient has no renal clearance. *Do not wait* until the creatinine reaches any specific number to say the patient has AKI. Any rise in creatinine indicates kidney injury.
- **Falling urine output** – The terms oliguria and anuria are used to describe a low urine output and no urine output respectively. In day-to-day practice these terms are not particularly useful, and it is more important to look for trends in urine output. In general, a urine output of less than 0.5 mL/kg/h is abnormally low.

It is important to remember that most patients with renal tract obstruction will have polyuria and not oliguria or anuria unless they develop complete obstruction, which is rare except in the context of acute surgical obstruction.

Key points

- Deterioration in vital signs should be recognised and reported promptly, particularly a fall in blood pressure and rising respiratory rate and pulse rate.
- A rise in creatinine of 50-100 µmol/L/day from baseline indicates severe kidney injury.
- Monitoring of urine output in acutely ill patients is essential. Urine output of less than 0.5 mL/kg/h must be reported.

Table 7.1 RIFLE classification for acute kidney injury.

Stage	Glomerular filtration rate (GFR) criteria	Urine output criteria
Risk	Creatinine increase×1.5 or GFR decrease >25%	<0.5 mL/kg/h×6 hours
Injury	Creatinine increase×2 or GFR decrease >50%	<0.5 mL/kg/h×12 hours
Failure	Creatinine increase×3 or GFR decrease >75% or serum creatinine >354	<0.3 mL/kg/h×24 hours or anuria×12 hours
Loss	Dialysis-dependent >4 weeks	
End-stage kidney disease	Dialysis-dependent >3 months	

Bellomo (2005) with permission from Elsevier.

Adverse consequences of kidney injury on hospital survival

In an Australian study of hospitalised patients identified by the RIFLE classification (Table 7.1), Uchino *et al.* (2010) demonstrated the serious consequences of either a transient (less than three-day) or more prolonged episode of AKI. Hospitalised patients who develop renal injury have a higher risk of death. Those with a transient rise in creatinine lasting less than three days had an inpatient mortality of 15%, and those with renal injury lasting greater than three days had an inpatient mortality of nearly 30%. Care could be improved by identifying at-risk individuals.

Risk factors for perioperative kidney injury

In the NCEPOD report *Adding Insult to Injury: Reviewing the Care of Patients who Died in Hospital With a Primary Diagnosis of Acute Kidney Injury* (2009), the authors reviewed 976 adult cases from over 200 NHS hospitals in the UK who had died in a three-month period. They found that over 20% of patients who developed AKI and subsequently died had 'forseeable and avoidable AKI'. Only 50% of patients were considered to have received a good standard of care. Failings were found in identification of 'at-risk' patients and in the management of AKI and its complications.

The care of patients at risk of AKI and of those with existing CKD can be improved by identifying them prior to problems arising. Opportunities to do this include:

- at the time of diagnosis of chronic medical conditions associated with CKD
- at the time of the prescription of medications that increase the risk of acute deterioration in kidney function with dehydration/hypovolaemia

- at the point of deciding to list for an operative procedure
- at pre-assessment for anaesthesia/operation
- at admission to hospital
- immediately preoperatively

Individuals who can be alerted to this increased risk include the patient, medical staff (including ward doctors, surgeons and anaesthetists) and nursing staff (including the pre-assessment clinic nurses, ward nurses, clinic nurses and theatre nurses). Patients who might be given specific warnings include those with pre-existing CKD, especially in the presence of other comorbidity such as heart failure or diabetes and those taking high-risk drugs including ACE inhibitors, angiotensin II receptor blockers (ARBs), direct renin inhibitors, diuretics, metformin and non-steroidal anti-inflammatory drugs (NSAIDs) (see Chapter 8). Patients may need both verbal and written information, such as clinic letters and information sheets.

Patients identified as at increased risk should then receive enhanced care on admission to hospital, whether for planned or emergency treatment.

Surgical patients

Patients admitted to the surgical ward might be highlighted to the medical team for review, or specifically to the renal team for review. This should occur *before* any further deterioration in renal function in the hope of avoiding acute-on-chronic kidney injury, rather than after the event. Patients requiring an operation might need pre-optimisation, with transfer to either HDU or ICU pre-operatively for optimisation of intravascular volume and cardiac output prior to surgery (Brienza *et al*. 2009). Patients likely to need HDU or ICU support postoperatively should have been identified prior to their operation. Patients who will be well enough to return to the general ward but who require enhanced surveillance can be identified to the critical care outreach team. Ward nurses should be made aware of the increased risk of kidney problems and the need for close monitoring and prompt reporting of any signs of deterioration.

Medical patients

Medical patients with or at risk of worsening renal injury should be highlighted to the renal team early in the course of their hospital admission. Critical care outreach, HDU and ICU should be involved early to pre-empt catastrophic deterioration on the general ward. Ward nurses caring for these patients must be made aware of the potential for deterioration and the action to take should this occur.

Key points

- AKI and acute-on-chronic kidney injury is often preventable.
- All staff involved in the patient's care must be made aware of increased risk in certain patients, including ward nurses, critical care outreach, HDU and ICU.
- Renal teams should be alerted to high-risk patients when they are admitted to hospital for both elective and emergency procedures.

Our index case

- 72 year old man
- PMH

  - Hypertension
  - Type 2 diabetes
  - Ischaemic heart disease
  - Osteoarthritis
  - CKD (eGFR 34 mL/min)

- Drug history
  - Metformin 500 mg tds
  - Gliclazide 80 mg bd
  - Enalapril 20 mg bd
  - Bendroflumethiazide 2.5 mg od
  - Atenolol 50 mg od

Risk factors?

Figure 7.1 Our index case.

Our index case

Examine the index case (Figure 7.1). We will return to this gentleman later in the chapter, but for now assume that he has had an orthopaedic operation under spinal anaesthetic. Read through his details and try to identify all the factors that put him at high risk for AKI and the time points at which they could have been identified.

Impact of surgery on kidney function

For the surgical patient the most important threat to the kidneys is a reduction in renal blood flow during the perioperative period. This may be due to either absolute (true) or relative hypovolaemia (Table 7.2). Absolute hypovolaemia reflects a decrease in absolute circulating volume. When blood volume falls, blood pressure is reduced and renal blood flow will fall. The normal response to a fall in renal blood flow is narrowing (constriction) of the post-glomerular efferent arteriole. This increases resistance to blood leaving the glomerulus and hence glomerular filtration is maintained (Figure 7.2). This efferent arteriolar constriction is dependent on angiotensin II, which is generated by the renin–angiotensin system (Figure 7.3). Angiotensinogen is cleaved by renin to form angiotensin I (blocked by renin inhibitors), which in turn is converted to angiotensin II by angiotensin converting enzyme (blocked by ACE inhibitors). Angiotensin II binds to angiotensin II receptors on the efferent arteriole, leading to vasoconstriction (blocked by angiotensin II receptor blockers, ARBs). Each of these groups of drugs will prevent the normal response to a fall in renal blood flow and so increase the risk of AKI if volume depletion occurs.

Volume depletion will be exacerbated by the use of diuretics, and hypotension by the use of other blood pressure lowering medication. Being 'nil by mouth' for a prolonged period of time will further exacerbate the risk of volume depletion.

Table 7.2 Causes of hypovolaemia.

Absolute hypovolaemia	Relative hypovolaemia
Haemorrhage	High cardiac output
GI losses (diarrhoea/vomiting)	• Sepsis
Skin losses (burns)	• Hepatorenal failure
Renal losses (polyuria)	Low cardiac output
	• Cardiac failure

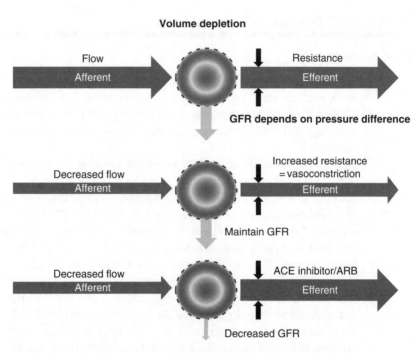

Figure 7.2 The intra-renal vascular response to volume depletion.

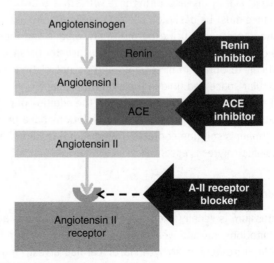

Figure 7.3 The renin–angiotensin system.

Key points

- The commonest cause of AKI in surgical patients is hypovolaemia leading to reduction in glomerular perfusion.
- Drugs that interfere with the renin–angiotensin system will increase the risk of hypovolaemia-induced AKI.

Impact of CKD on standard protocols

Fluid management

Perioperative fluid regimes are designed to maintain euvolaemia. The traditional postoperative 3-litre fluid regime (typically 2L of 5% dextrose/1L of 0.9% sodium chloride) may need modifying in patients with kidney disease. In addition, the GIFTASUP recommendations (Powell-Tuck et al. 2006) need to be considered.

Daily fluid requirements need to be individualised to each patient. A patient recovering from kidney injury may be polyuric with a very high urine output and need several litres of fluid a day. An anuric dialysis-dependent patient may need less than 1000 mL of fluid per day. A patient with CKD may fall anywhere between these two extremes, and care needs to be taken to avoid giving too little fluid, leading to hypovolaemia and worsening pre-renal kidney injury, or giving too much fluid, leading to peripheral and pulmonary oedema.

The sodium content of fluid will also need to be individualised. 0.9% sodium chloride solution is actually hypertonic, containing 154 mmol sodium per litre. The more physiologically balanced fluids recommended in GIFTASUP have a lower sodium and chloride content (and therefore closer to physiologic). However, they also have a fixed potassium content. There is little published experience assessing their use in patients with acute, acute-on-chronic or chronic kidney disease, or in those with stage 5 CKD. Daily assessment of fluid balance must be based on clinical examination (pulse, blood pressure, jugular venous pressure), urine output, daily weight and input/output charts. Daily weights are the best guide to changes in water balance, but can sometimes be difficult to obtain in ill patients and do not distinguish between fluid in the vascular space and fluid in the interstitial space.

Particular care must be taken with the addition of potassium to intravenous fluid. Some intravenous crystalloid solutions have pre-added potassium (e.g. Hartmann's solution contains 5 mmol/L potassium). Daily assessment of urea and electrolytes is essential.

Hyperkalaemia

Potassium is renally excreted. Hyperkalaemia may cause symptoms such as palpitations, muscle weakness or paralysis. However, the first symptom may be life-threatening arrhythmia or cardiac arrest, and hyperkalaemia is one of the commonest causes of sudden death in patients with kidney failure.

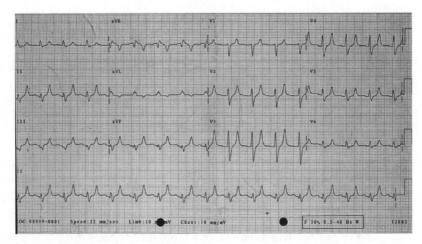

Figure 7.4 Hyperkalaemia: peaking of T wave and widening of QRS complex.

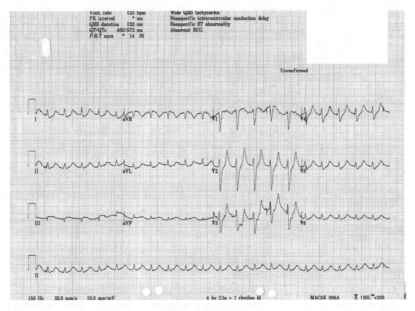

Figure 7.5 Hyperkalaemia: peaking of T wave, widening of QRS complex, loss of P wave.

Hyperkalaemia may be suspected from the electrocardiogram before the serum potassium is available. Conversely, if serum potassium is >6.5 mmol/L an ECG monitor should be attached to look for evidence of cardiac toxicity. Changes of hyperkalaemia include peaking of the T wave (Figure 7.4) , widening of the QRS complex (Figure 7.5), loss of the P wave (Figure 7.5), very broad QRS merging into the T wave (Figure 7.6) and a sine wave (Figure 7.7). If hyperkalaemia is suspected from the ECG, an arterial blood gas sample may allow a 'quick' result to guide urgent management.

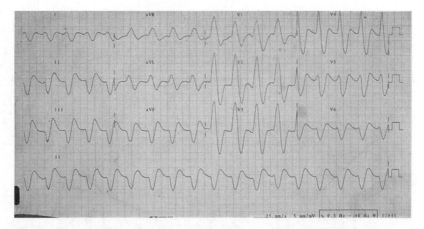

Figure 7.6 Hyperkalaemia: very broad QRS complex merging into the T wave.

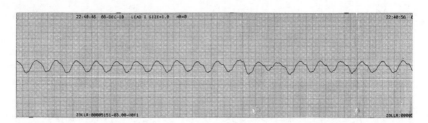

Figure 7.7 A sine wave.

Table 7.3 Causes of hyperkalaemia.

Exogenous potassium administration	Potassium redistribution	Reduced potassium excretion
Oral potassium supplements (Food)	Insulin deficiency Starvation (nil by mouth)	Volume depletion Spironolactone
Dioralyte	Beta-blockers	Amiloride
Stored blood	Post-dialysis rebound	ACE inhibitors
IV potassium		Angiotensin II receptor blockers
Which intravenous fluid?		Beta-blockers
		NSAIDs
		Trimethoprim
		Heparin

High potassium may be due to excessive potassium intake, potassium redistribution or reduced potassium excretion (Table 7.3). In contrast to popular belief, severe hyperkalaemia is rarely due to patient indiscretion, and advice to 'stop eating bananas' is rarely helpful. The management of acute severe hyperkalaemia is beyond the scope of this chapter.

Diabetes management

Many hospitals will use a standard prescription chart to manage patients with insulin-treated diabetes perioperatively. A typical regime includes 5% dextrose with potassium and soluble insulin (GKI). This regime may need altering in patients with impaired potassium excretion (omit potassium from the prescription) or who are fluid restricted (use a lower volume of a higher-concentration glucose solution, e.g. 500 mL of 10% dextrose in place of 1000 mL of 5% glucose).

Nutrition

Patients with acute, acute-on-chronic, chronic or end-stage kidney disease all have complex nutritional needs. They are frequently in a hypercatabolic state and are at high risk of malnutrition. Inappropriate dietary restriction is well meant, but misguided advice may exacerbate these potential problems. All will need assessment and support from specialist dietitians with experience in the management of patients with kidney disease (See Chapter 9).

Special considerations

Radiology contrast media (gadolinium/iodinated contrast)

Many patients admitted to hospital need further complex investigations to reach a diagnosis. The use of intravenous contrast-enhanced diagnostic imaging is common practice. Unfortunately intravenous iodinated contrast media have the potential to be nephrotoxic, and this potential is greatest in those with pre-existing kidney injury. Acute-on-chronic kidney injury secondary to contrast media is called contrast nephropathy, and it lengthens hospital stay, increases the need for dialysis and increases mortality. The risk of contrast nephropathy can be reduced by adequate pre-hydration, although it is unclear whether or not isotonic bicarbonate (1.26% sodium bicarbonate) is superior to saline (either 0.45% or 0.9% sodium chloride) (Brar et al. 2008). The addition of oral N-acetylcysteine may reduce the risk further with minimal toxicity (Kelly et al. 2008). Loop diuretics may be harmful and should be avoided (Kelly et al. 2008). Contrast nephropathy is both predictable and potentially avoidable, and therefore all hospitals should have mechanisms in place to identify at-risk individuals prior to administration of intravenous contrast. Once identified, protocol-driven practice should minimise the risk of contrast nephropathy.

Gadolinium is a contrast agent used in magnetic resonance imaging. Reports have linked gadolinium to the development of a rare but devastating condition called nephrogenic systemic fibrosis (NSF) in patients with advanced kidney failure (at least stage 4, but predominantly dialysis-treated stage 5 CKD: Nortier & del Marmol 2007). NSF can lead to both severe disability and mortality. Unlike contrast nephropathy, there is no effective strategy to mitigate the risk of developing NSF following gadolinium exposure, leading to a recommendation of avoidance unless the benefits of exposure outweigh the potential risk. More recently, evidence has emerged that the risk of NSF is not equal with all forms of gadolinium, and the Medicines and Healthcare products Regulatory Authority has offered guidance on which forms of gadolinium may be safer if exposure is required (MHRA 2010).

Bleeding (uraemic platelet dysfunction)

Patients with advanced CKD have an acquired disorder of platelet function. This leads to a prolonged bleeding time. This is rarely a clinical issue, but if prolonged bleeding occurs the bleeding time can be corrected by the administration of the synthetic vasopressin analogue desmopressin (DDAVP) at a dose of 0.4 µg/kg over 30 minutes. In our experience, excessive bleeding most commonly occurs due to over-heparinisation, and it always sensible to measure the activated partial thromboplastin time (aPTT) and prothrombin time (PT) first and correct these if abnormal. Desmopressin has been most useful in uraemic patients undergoing endoscopic retrograde cholangiopan-creatography (ERCP) and sphincterotomy, where we encountered significant bleeding prior to the prophylactic use of desmopressin and none since.

Medication management

As with any patient, a careful review of current and planned medication is essential in all patients at risk of AKI or with existing CKD. Specific concerns are:

(1) Plan to withdraw any medication that impairs maintenance of glomerular filtration rate (GFR) preoperatively. This should include ACE inhibitors and ARBs, which should be stopped at least 24 hours preoperatively unless there is a compelling reason to continue them.

(2) Plan to withdraw any medication that causes dehydration preoperatively. This should include diuretics, which should be discontinued on the day of surgery unless there is a compelling reason to continue them. For example, it would be reasonable to stop a thiazide that has been pre-scribed for hypertension, but you would be more concerned about stop-ping a loop diuretic that has been prescribed for heart failure.

(3) Review the need for any antihypertensive medication. If the patient will be nil by mouth or at risk of perioperative hypotension, then do they need to continue all of their antihypertensive medication? This will depend on current blood pressure, the type of blood pressure medication and the nature of the surgery. In general it might be sensible to discontinue a dihydropyridine calcium antagonist (e.g. nifedipine) in a patient having major abdominal surgery, but unreasonable to stop a beta-blocker (beta-blockers may reduce perioperative mortality, and acute withdrawal may lead to side effects).

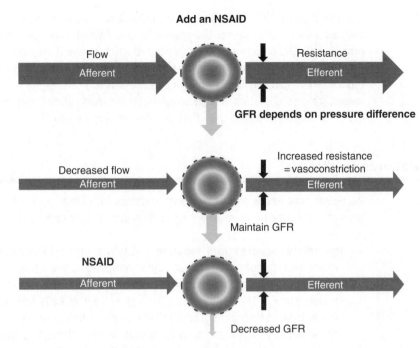

Figure 7.8 Effect of NSAIDs on glomerular filtration.

(4) Look for and discontinue nephrotoxic drugs. The obvious medications to look for are NSAIDs, which constrict the afferent arteriole, directly reducing GFR (Figure 7.8).
(5) Check for drugs that are renally excreted. Are they prescribed at the correct dose for the patient's current kidney function? If kidney function worsens, does the dose need to be reduced further? Good examples of drugs that accumulate and cause significant toxicity in renal failure include aciclovir (neurotoxicity), morphine/codeine metabolites (drowsiness, respiratory failure), gabapentin/pregabalin (drowsiness) and cephalosporins (neurotoxicity).
(6) Avoid prescribing new drugs that fall into the following categories:
   (a) Nephrotoxins – NSAIDs, antibiotics (particularly gentamicin and vancomycin). If gentamicin or vancomycin cannot be avoided it is imperative that blood levels are closely monitored to avoid toxic effects.
   (b) Analgesics that accumulate – opioids whose metabolites are renally excreted (morphine/codeine).
   (c) Drugs that cause hyperkalaemia – trimethoprim (which will also raise serum creatinine), potassium-sparing diuretics (amiloride, spironolactone).

Analgesia

Analgesics that accumulate in renal failure include opioids such as morphine, diamorphine and codeine. While these drugs are hepatically metabolised, their metabolites are renally excreted. These metabolites do not provide effective analgesia, but do cause drowsiness and respiratory depression.

Alternative opioids that show less accumulation include fentanil, alfentanil, methadone and oxycodone. Gabapentin and pregabalin also accumulate in renal failure and require significant dose reduction to avoid toxicity.

NSAIDs cause afferent arteriolar vasoconstriction and will predictably reduce GFR, especially in the presence of pre-existing CKD, heart failure, liver failure, volume depletion and in patients taking medications that block the action of angiotensin II on the efferent arteriole (Figure 7.8).

Patients on dialysis

Particular care needs to be taken with patients with stage 5 CKD treated by dialysis during the perioperative period. Specific areas to look out for include:

(1) **Post-dialysis potassium rebound** – Patients with no kidney function cannot excrete potassium. Potassium is removed during a haemodialysis treatment, but then progressively accumulates until the next dialysis session. Most of the body potassium is stored within cells and not in the bloodstream. So serum potassium falls quickly on dialysis as we dialyse the blood, but increases again immediately post dialysis as potassium moves out of the cells and into the bloodstream (Figure 7.9). This is called potassium rebound. It is important not to be 'fooled' by a low potassium immediately after dialysis. Repeat the potassium 1-2 hours later and it will usually have risen back into the normal range. Administering intravenous potassium immediately post-dialysis risks precipitating severe hyperkalaemia.

(2) **Nil by mouth** – 'Starvation' can lead to relative hypoinsulinaemia, resulting in an extracellular potassium shift and increasing serum potassium. This can be avoided by prescribing 500 mL of 10% glucose over 12 hours in dialysis patients who will be kept nil by mouth overnight preoperatively. Urea and electrolytes should be taken 1-2 hours after surgery to check for hyperkalaemia.

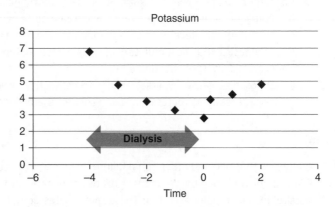

Figure 7.9 Potassium levels pre and post dialysis (potassium rebound).

(3) **Preservation of veins** – Patients with stage 5 CKD will need renal replacement therapy (RRT) for the rest of their lives. For some this will be a kidney transplant, but many rely on dialysis as a life-prolonging treatment. These patients depend on access to the venous circulation for their dialysis treatment. Ideally this should be by using a peripheral forearm vein connected to the radial artery for a forearm fistula. If this fails then we would move to the upper arm (cephalic) vein connected to the brachial artery. To allow long-term dialysis, healthcare professionals need to try and preserve their patients' veins (and arteries) by avoiding unnecessary venepuncture and cannulation. In a patient with advanced CKD, the renal team will usually have identified the best site for an arterio-venous fistula, and it is important that this site is protected during hospital admission. Wherever possible, use the veins in the back of the hand for venous cannulae, as this will not cause damage for future fistula formation.

Central veins can also be damaged by central venous cannulation. This can lead to stenosis and diminished flow or even occlusion (Figure 7.10). This will compromise the chance of a fistula working in the long-term. Central stenoses are more common with subclavian than jugular lines, and jugular lines may be preferable in patients at risk of AKI or with established CKD.

Some patients may be admitted with a functioning arteriovenous fistula or arteriovenous graft (a piece of synthetic tubing tunnelled under the

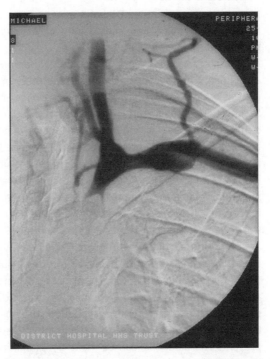

Figure 7.10 Central venous occlusion proximal to the left subclavian and internal jugular veins.

skin between an artery and vein - usually in the arm or upper leg). It is important that these sites are not used for blood pressure measurements, venepuncture or cannulation. This is to protect the site from damage, but also because bleeding will occur at near arterial pressure from a fistula/graft. The patient should be given an 'alert' wristband to wear on the fistula limb, to alert staff of its presence.

There is also a risk of a fistula or graft clotting if the patient becomes hypovolaemic/hypotensive postoperatively. Checks should be made for the presence of a 'thrill' (buzzing sensation) and bruit using a stethoscope. Absence of a thrill or bruit should be reported to the renal team as soon as possible.

(4) **Dialysis access lines** - Some patients undergoing haemodialysis will have either temporary or permanent venous access catheters to allow access to their venous blood for dialysis. These lines are usually placed in the jugular, femoral or, rarely, subclavian veins. They may consist of a single line with two lumens, or two separate lines with a single lumen each. Temporary lines enter the vein at the site of skin puncture. Permanent lines are tunnelled under the skin prior to entering the vein in a manner similar to a Hickman line used for chemotherapy or parenteral nutrition.

The major problems encountered with dialysis access lines are thrombosis and infection. Because of the high frequency of thrombosis the lines are often 'locked' with a high concentration of heparin. The line locking solution should never be flushed into the patient, as this can cause systemic anticoagulation. **Dialysis access lines should not be used for any other purpose, and should only be accessed by dialysis trained personnel**.

Line infection is a major complication of haemodialysis, contributing to a significant morbidity and increased mortality in this patient group. Any dialysis patient with a dialysis line who becomes unwell should be assumed to have line sepsis until proven otherwise. Blood cultures should be obtained from the line and from a peripheral vein as soon as possible and antibiotics commenced to cover *Staphylococcus aureus* (the commonest line pathogen) pending culture results. The exit site may also be a site for infection, and should be assessed in the case of pyrexia or other signs of infection. Swabs should be taken if the site is inflamed and/or any exudate is present.

(5) **Peritoneal dialysis patients** - Approximately 20% of dialysis patients are on peritoneal dialysis rather than haemodialysis. These patients have a permanent plastic catheter placed into their abdominal cavity through their anterior abdominal wall. They may present to the surgical ward with a unique form of peritonitis complicating their dialysis treatment. Their peritonitis presents with severe abdominal pain, guarding and rebound tenderness in the same way that a patient with surgical peritonitis would present. The diagnosis can be made by examining a sample of the peritoneal dialysis fluid, which is usually collected by one of the peritoneal dialysis nurses. The sample will look cloudy to the naked eye. When

examined in the microbiology laboratory, it contains >100 white blood cells per $100/mm^3$ and bacteria may be seen on a Gram-stained film. Peritonitis can occur through an exit site infection (inflammation/pus around the site where the catheter leaves the abdominal wall), contamination of the peritoneal dialysis catheter, dialysis fluid or the connection between the dialysis system and the catheter. The infection can usually be treated with antibiotics that are added to the peritoneal dialysis fluid. Occasionally a peritoneal dialysis patient will develop an acute surgical abdomen in the same way that any other person can. Important clues to this are mixed organisms on culture (suggesting large bowel perforation), persistent symptoms despite standard treatment, bile-stained dialysis fluid (suggesting biliary perforation) and faecal contamination (suggesting large bowel perforation).

(6) **Blood transfusion** – Blood transfusion raises additional concerns in patients on dialysis. Most dialysis patients have chronic anaemia secondary to erythropoietin deficiency, and many will be treated with synthetic erythropoietins. These will lose their efficacy rapidly during any acute illness, and haemoglobin will fall quickly. Most patients will tolerate this well, and transfusion should be used for particular indications and not simply because the haemoglobin is 'low'.

Specific concerns about transfusing stored blood include the fluid volume, the potassium content and the risk of sensitisation to human leucocyte antigens. In an anuric dialysis patient who is not acutely bleeding, it is safer to transfuse on dialysis to avoid the risk of volume overload and/or pulmonary oedema. The extracellular potassium content of stored blood is highly variable, depending on how long it has been stored, and it can be as high as 40 mmol/L. Again it is safer to transfuse when the patient is dialysing to avoid the risk of acute hyperkalaemia.

One of the major barriers to successful renal transplantation is the presence of antibodies to human leucocyte antigens. This means that a patient has previously been exposed to 'foreign' antigens on another person's cells, which restricts the chances of getting a kidney transplant. Multiple blood transfusions are one of the main reasons behind the development of these antibodies.

Renal transplant patients

Renal transplant patients now represent the largest group of patients receiving long-term RRT. All kidney transplant patients are on medication to prevent transplant rejection, most have abnormal kidney function (i.e. reduced GFR) and most have hypertension treated with medication, including drugs that inhibit angiotensin II. They are therefore at high risk of AKI both through mechanisms unique to a kidney transplant (e.g. acute rejection, surgical complications of the renal artery or ureteric anastomosis) or through mechanisms common to any patient, most commonly pre-renal kidney injury.

(1) **Immunosuppressive medication** needs to be continued during hospital admission. Ciclosporin and tacrolimus are available in different preparations with different bioavailability. Patients should be prescribed their usual brand of medication to avoid sudden changes in drug levels. If a patient is nil by mouth, oral prednisolone can be converted to intravenous hydrocortisone in the short term. Both ciclosporin and tacrolimus can be given intravenously, but you should liaise with a specialist pharmacist to ensure appropriate dose conversion. Drug levels will need to be carefully monitored. It is usually safe to discontinue azathioprine or mycophenolate in the short term if a patient is required to be nil by mouth.

(2) **Steroids** – In the acutely unwell patient it may be necessary to increase the steroid dose to avoid an acute Addisonian crisis, especially in patients who have received long-term steroids. One overlooked concern is the potential for steroids to mask the acute abdomen. We have seen patients present with minimal abdominal signs despite intra-abdominal pathologies including gangrenous appendix, multiple colonic perforations secondary to cytomegalovirus (CMV) colitis and faecal peritonitis secondary to perforated diverticular disease. In any chronically immunosuppressed patient presenting with abdominal symptoms/signs that do not settle, there should be a low threshold for further investigation or even laparotomy.

Conservative care

An increasing number of patients with advanced kidney failure are electing for conservative care rather than dialysis as their preferred treatment pathway. This decision needs careful documentation in the case notes. Even with careful documentation, the implications may not be explicit (Box 7.1).

Scenarios

It is time to return to our index case (Figure 7.1). This gentleman does indeed have a number of risk factors for AKI, as shown in Figure 7.11. The following sections place him in three different scenarios and consider the management issues in each case.

Acute gout

The patient (our index case: Figures 7.1, 7.11) asks to see the ward doctor because of severe pain in his right great toe. The pain came on during the night two days after knee surgery for a left total knee replacement. The pain is very severe and the patient thinks he has gout – at least that's what he was told two years ago when he had similar symptoms. He wants to know what can be done to control his symptoms as quickly as possible. Outline a plan of management.

Box 7.1   Case study

An 88-year-old woman with multiple medical comorbidities was seen in the renal clinic with an estimated GFR (eGFR) of 12 mL/min. This was thought to be due to hypertension and ischaemic nephropathy on the background of extensive vascular disease. Following extensive discussion with the renal multidisciplinary team and her family, the patient decided that she did not wish to undergo dialysis should the need arise in the future. A conservative care package was put in place, including nursing home support. Over the next few months her eGFR fell to 9 mL/min and her overall quality of life decreased, necessitating nursing home admission. All of this was documented in her medical notes.

Shortly after being admitted to the nursing home she fell and fractured her neck of femur. She was admitted to hospital. At admission her eGFR was 7 mL/min. In keeping with the care pathway for fractured neck of femur she had early surgical repair. Postoperatively her eGFR was 5 mL/min and she was referred for renal support. At this stage the patient was too drowsy to take an active part in decision making, and following review of the case notes and discussion between the renal team and her family, the patient was transferred to a palliative care pathway and died comfortably within 48 hours.

On review it was felt that this lady had undergone an unnecessary surgical intervention and could have been managed conservatively throughout her admission.

Our index case – risk factors

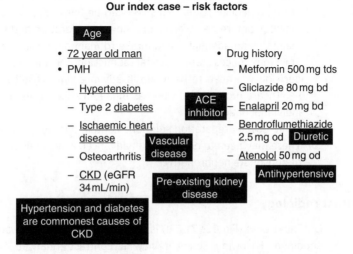

Figure 7.11 Our index case (Figure 7.1) with risk factors for AKI highlighted.

(1) Ideally confirm the diagnosis. This should include the exclusion of other diagnoses – especially septic arthritis. A definite diagnosis would require aspiration of fluid from the joint both for microscopy, sensitivity and culture to exclude septic arthritis and for microscopy for negatively birefringent crystals to confirm gout. Serum uric acid levels may be elevated, but this is unhelpful as they are nearly always elevated in patients with chronic kidney disease.

(2) Provide effective analgesia. The usual first-line analgesic for acute gout is an NSAID. Unfortunately they are contraindicated in this case. Alternatives include oral colchicine or oral or intramuscular steroid. Oral colchicine is effective, but the dose is limited by diarrhoea which could cause volume depletion and precipitate acute-on-chronic kidney injury. Oral prednisolone at a dose of 20–30 mg per day for 7–10 days or a single intramuscular injection of kenalog at a dose of 80 mg is usually effective with a low risk of side effects in the absence of a contraindication.

(3) Prevention of recurrence. This is a longer-term management issue and will involve liaison between the patient, the primary care physician and possibly the renal team.

Colonoscopy

Our index case (Figures 7.1, 7.11) has been referred for investigation of unexplained iron deficiency anaemia. He requires a colonoscopy. What advice would you offer?

(1) This patient is at significant risk of electrolyte imbalance and acute-on-chronic kidney injury when receiving bowel preparation for colonoscopy. These risks have been highlighted by the National Patient Safety Agency (2009). All healthcare organisations should have an appropriate system in place to minimise this risk.

(2) The risk of AKI is predominantly secondary to volume depletion leading to pre-renal kidney failure. This risk can be minimised by stopping his ACE inhibitor before he receives oral bowel preparation and ensuring that he maintains an adequate fluid intake to maintain his intravascular volume. This may necessitate hospital admission for intravenous fluids. This decision will need to be made in advance on a case-by-case basis by a healthcare professional who has made an appropriate assessment of the individual patient.

(3) Some bowel preparation solutions contain a large quantity of phosphate. These may need to be avoided in advanced kidney failure to avoid the risk of phosphate nephropathy.

Contrast radiology

Our index case (Figures 7.1, 7.11) is admitted to the surgical ward with an acute abdomen. Following senior review a contrast-enhanced CT scan of the abdomen is requested. What advice would you offer?

(1) This patient is at risk of contrast nephropathy.
(2) While the evidence base is not conclusive on the best form of intravenous fluid to use, there is good evidence that adequate pre-hydration decreases the risk of contrast nephropathy. The use of 0.45% sodium chloride or 1.26% (isotonic) sodium bicarbonate probably offers the greatest benefit, with a lower risk of fluid overload in comparison to 0.9% sodium chloride.
(3) Oral N-acetylcysteine (Parvolex) at a dose of 600 mg twice a day for 48 hours may further reduce the risk of contrast nephropathy. While the evidence of benefit has been conflicting, there is no evidence of harm and there is minimal additional cost to this treatment. Other adjuncts (furosemide and aminophylline) have not shown consistent benefit and may in fact be harmful.

Intravenous hydration only needs to commence one hour prior to the CT and does not need to delay his investigation unduly. Hydration should then continue until six hours post-procedure. As with all procedures, a judgement has to be made as to the balance between the urgency of proceeding with investigation and treatment and the need to take due care to avoid any unnecessary and avoidable harm that might arise from them.

Conclusion

Anyone can suffer acute kidney injury in hospital, even if they have no history of kidney problems. However, people with pre-existing kidney impairment are particularly vulnerable to further kidney damage during the course of a hospital stay. Kidney function can worsen through a number of factors including nephrotoxic medication, dehydration and/or low blood pressure.

Patients with stage 5 CKD treated by either dialysis or kidney transplantation, who are admitted to hospital for other reasons, should usually be jointly managed with the renal team.

Patients with end-stage kidney disease who have elected for conservative management of their kidney failure should be clearly identified. This may minimise the chances of undertaking unnecessary interventions at the end of life.

In all cases, standard operating protocols should be available that include advice on how to identify people at risk of acute or acute-on-chronic kidney injury, manage any deterioration in kidney function and avoid any predictable complications in patients with established disease. Proactive and anticipatory management of these issues can improve patient outcomes and prevent avoidable escalations of care. The renal team are a useful resource in managing patients with kidney disease regardless of the healthcare setting.

Take-home messages

● Identify patients at risk of acute or acute-on-chronic kidney injury early.
● Withdraw unnecessary medication and pre-optimise patients before they go to theatre.

- Use critical care outreach.
- Don't ignore small rises in serum creatinine – they indicate significant kidney injury.
- Patients on RRT (dialysis or transplant) need special consideration regarding management when admitted to hospital for other reasons.

References

Bellomo, R. (2005) Defining, quantifying, and classifying acute renal failure. *Critical Care Clinics*, **21**, 223–37.

Brar, S.S., Yuh-Jer Shen, A., Jorgensen, M.B. *et al.* (2008) Sodium bicarbonate vs sodium chloride for the prevention of contrast medium-induced nephropathy in patients undergoing coronary angiography. *JAMA*, **300**, 1038–46.

Brienza, T., Giglio, M.T., Marucci, M., Fiore, T. (2009) Does perioperative hemody-namic optimization protect renal function in surgical patients? A meta-analytic study. *Critical Care Medicine*, **37**, 2079–90.

Kelly, A.M., Dwamena, B., Cronin, P., Bernstein, S.J. & Carlos, R.C. (2008) Meta-analysis: effectiveness of drugs for preventing contrast-induced nephropathy. *Annals of Internal Medicine*, **148**, 284–94.

MHRA (2010) Gadolinium-containing contrast agents: new advice to minimise the risk of nephrogenic systemic fibrosis. Drug safety update. http://www.mhra.gov.uk/Safetyinformation/DrugSafetyUpdate/CON087741 (accessed September 2012).

National Patient Safety Agency (2009) Reducing risk of harm from oral bowel cleansing solutions. NPSA Rapid Response Report NPSA/2009/RRR012. http://www.nrls.npsa.nhs.uk/resources/type/alerts/?entryid45=59869&p=2 (accessed September 2012).

NCEPOD (2009) *Adding Insult to Injury: Reviewing the Care of Patients who Died in Hospital With a Primary Diagnosis of Acute Kidney Injury*. http://www.ncepod.org.uk/2009aki.htm (accessed September 2012).

Nortier, J.L. & del Marmol, V. (2007) Nephrogenic systemic fibrosis: the need for a multidisciplinary approach. *Nephrology, Dialysis, Transplantation*, **22**, 3097–101.

Powell-Tuck, J., Gosling, P., Lobo, D.N. *et al.* (2006) *British Consensus Guidelines on Intravenous Fluid Therapy for Adult Surgical Patients* (GIFTASUP). http://www.bapen.org.uk/pdfs/bapen_pubs/giftasup.pdf (accessed September 2012).

Stevens, P.E., O'Donoghue, D.J., de Lusignan, S. *et al.* (2007) Chronic kidney disease management in the United Kingdom: NEOERICA project results. *Kidney International*, **72**, 92–9.

Uchino, S., Bellomo, R., Bagshaw, S.M., *et al.* (2010) Transient azotaemia is associated with a high risk of death in hospitalized patients. *Nephrology, Dialysis, Transplantation*, **25**, 1833–9.

Chapter 8

Medication Management and Chronic Kidney Disease

Aileen Dunleavy

Crosshouse Hospital, Kilmarnock, UK

Introduction

Medication management in patients with chronic kidney disease (CKD) is often complex, and whilst regimes are adjusted to accommodate individual health states and treatment modalities, they are usually guided by some general principles. Safe and effective prescribing for people with CKD requires some basic knowledge of the patient's condition, including the degree of renal impairment, whether the patient is receiving renal replacement therapy (RRT) and if so what type, and whether the patient has any residual urine output. In addition, some understanding of the pharmacokinetics of the drugs being prescribed is important. Whilst medication management for patients with stage 4–5 kidney disease is largely managed by a nephrologist and a specialist pharmacist, patients are often admitted to other services and treated in primary care. Most renal services provide prescribing advice and support for patients receiving care in non-specialist areas. In addition, the *Renal Drug Handbook* (Ashley & Currie 2009) is available electronically and in hardback and is widely used, both within specialist services and increasingly within others. Ongoing communication within and between primary and secondary care providers is an important part of ensuring safe and effective medication management for people with CKD.

Measurement of renal impairment

There is limited information in the *British National Formulary* (BNF) and from drug manufacturers about dosing in patients with renal impairment, and it is best to use sources such as the local renal unit or the *Renal Drug Handbook*, which is widely used in specialist renal units and is based on licensing information, case studies, research papers and expert opinion.

Kidney Disease Management: A Practical Approach for the Non-Specialist Healthcare Practitioner, First Edition. Edited by Rachel Lewis and Helen Noble.
© 2013 John Wiley & Sons, Ltd. Published 2013 by John Wiley & Sons, Ltd.

When advising on dosage adjustments it is important to know:

- how the drug is handled by the body, e.g. whether it is renally excreted
- if the drug has a narrow therapeutic index, e.g. digoxin
- what side effects are to be expected
- the severity of the condition being treated

Previously creatinine clearance was used as a measure of renal function, but this is not a good marker, especially in patients with a low body mass, and therefore many patients with CKD were not identified. The Modification of Diet in Renal Disease (MDRD) equation was introduced in 2002 as a means of measuring estimated glomerular filtration rate (eGFR) and was validated in Caucasian and African-American CKD patients. It takes into account creatinine, age, sex and some racial groups and has been normalised for a body surface area of $1.73\,m^2$. eGFR is now reported from all laboratories in the UK at the same time as creatinine clearance, with the result that it is now easier to recognise patients with renal impairment. eGFR is a sufficiently accurate indication of renal impairment for most patients and the majority of drugs. As most manufacturers studies used Cockcroft Gault this should be used for high-risk drugs with narrow therapeutic ranges, oncology drugs and nephrotoxic agents.

Cockcroft and Gault equation

$$\text{Creatinine clearance}\,(\text{mL/min}) = \frac{(140 - \text{age}) \times \text{weight}\,(\text{kg})}{\text{serum creatinine}\,(\mu\,\text{mol/L})} \times F$$

where $F = 1.23$ (males), 1.04 (females).

Ideal body weight should be used for obese patients, as actual bodyweight would overestimate creatinine clearance, leading to an overdose. Actual bodyweight should be used for heavy muscle-bound patients to prevent underdosing. Table 8.1 shows some limitations and inaccuracies of the Cockcroft & Gault and MDRD equations.

Table 8.1 Limitations and inaccuracies of the equations.

Cockcroft & Gault (creatinine clearance, mL/min)	MDRD (eGFR, mL/min/1.73 m²)
People in catabolic states	Transplant patients
Extensive oedema	Serious comorbidities, e.g. diabetes
Certain races	Certain races
Rapidly changing renal function	Extremes or rapidly changing renal function
Extremes of body weight	Extremes of body weight
Pregnant women	Pregnant women
Increased creatine consumption	Increased creatine consumption
Children	Children

Principles of drug dosing in renal impairment

Various pharmacokinetic factors are altered in kidney disease, and renal replacement therapy (RRT) can alter the excretion of some medication. Many drugs are renally excreted or have renally excreted metabolites, leading to a need for dosage adjustments in patients with renal impairment.

The main pharmacokinetic parameters that may be altered in CKD are:

- bioavailability
- distribution
- metabolism
- elimination

Bioavailability

Bioavailability is defined as the percentage of an administered drug that reaches the systemic circulation. In the case of oral administration, it is the percentage of the drug that is absorbed across the gastrointestinal membrane. Intravenous drugs have 100% bioavailability, but the bioavailability of drugs administered by other routes may vary considerably with drug, formulation and individual patient. Altered bioavailability can lead to erratic absorption and enhanced adverse drug reactions.

Renal impairment can affect absorption by:

- Altered gastrointestinal motility – Absorption is reduced by nausea, vomiting, diarrhoea, peritonitis or oedema, e.g. reduced availability of furosemide in oedematous patients.
- Increased gastric pH due to increased blood urea nitrogen levels and the majority of CKD patients being on stomach protection, e.g. H_2-antagonists (ranitidine) or proton-pump inhibitors (omeprazole, lansoprazole). Some medication is best absorbed in acidic conditions, so if the gastric pH is too high it can lead to reduced absorption e.g. ferrous sulphate.
- Reduced absorption due to insoluble chelate formation, e.g. drug interactions between phosphate binders and iron tablets.

Distribution

After a drug is administered it disperses throughout the body until it reaches equilibrium. This is called the apparent volume of distribution (V_d), which is a ratio of the amount of drug in the body to the amount of the drug in the plasma. Drugs are distributed into areas with the highest blood flow first. A low V_d is seen with highly protein-bound or water-soluble drugs. A high V_d is seen with fat-soluble or un-ionised drugs due to increased tissue penetration.

In renal failure this can be altered by:

- Hydration – V_d of water-soluble drugs is increased if the patient is oedematous or has ascites, and conversely in dehydrated patients the V_d may be reduced.
- Reduced protein binding, due to uraemia changing the shape of binding sites, drugs or waste products competing for binding sites, inadequate nutrition causing low albumin levels, inflammation or dialysis, especially peritoneal dialysis. Highly protein-bound drugs are most affected.
- Changes in tissue binding – This is rarely of clinical importance apart from in the case of digoxin, where the V_d can be reduced by up to 50%, so that patients with CKD stages 3–5 require a reduced loading dose.

Hydration and reduced protein binding are usually only clinically relevant in drugs with narrow therapeutic indexes and low V_d (less than 0.7 L/kg), e.g. theophylline, and can result in an increased V_d and toxicity.

An important example is phenytoin, where binding is reduced if GFR is less than 25 mL/min or if the patient has low albumin levels (<4.4 g/dL). This causes increased concentrations of free drug. This is critical when interpreting phenytoin drug levels, as the measured level will be falsely low and should be adjusted.

Metabolism

This usually occurs in the liver to make drugs more water-soluble so that they can be more easily excreted. Some drugs are metabolised in the kidney to their active form, e.g. vitamin D, or to renally excreted active metabolites, e.g. morphine and pethidine. This can lead to the adverse effects and toxicity seen with some medication due to accumulation. The metabolic pathways of reduction and hydrolysis are reduced in renal impairment.

In CKD, metabolism can also be increased, as more drug is available for metabolism due to reduced protein binding and uraemic toxins inducing hepatic enzymes.

Elimination

The elimination half-life ($T_{1/2}$) is the time taken for free drug concentrations in the body to halve. The renal excretion of medication depends on glomerular filtration, active tubular excretion and passive tubular reabsorption. In renal failure, if a drug is renally excreted its $T_{1/2}$ will be increased. This can affect the dose and frequency of administration of medication: for example, the $T_{1/2}$ of gentamicin is increased from 1–3 hours to over 24 hours, so it only has to be given every 48 hours to CKD 5 patients.

If a dose adjustment is required, either reduce the dose or increase the dosage interval. The option used will depend on the dosage units available and what would be most convenient for the patient and nursing staff. If high serum drug concentrations are needed quickly then loading doses may be required due to reduced absorption and increased $T_{1/2}$, as it takes longer to reach steady state ($5 \times T_{1/2}$).

In CKD and haemodialysis some physiological actions can be altered, and this can contribute either to enhanced effects or to increased adverse drug reactions:

- Hypovolaemia or haemodialysis (if the patient has put on too much weight between sessions, requiring rapid removal of excess fluid during dialysis) can lead to an enhanced blood-pressure-lowering effect with antihypertensives.
- Increased risk of hyperkalaemia with angiotensin converting enzyme inhibitors (ACE inhibitors) or angiotensin receptor blockers (ARBs), potassium-sparing diuretics and potassium salts.
- Uraemia can cause excess bleeding with antiplatelets or anticoagulants.
- Enhanced CNS sensitivity to centrally acting drugs, e.g. antidepressants, analgesics (especially opioids), medication for neuropathic pain, e.g. gabapentin.
- Electrolyte variations, e.g. digoxin toxicity due to potassium shifts pre and post dialysis.

Patients with CKD are usually prescribed medication for life, but their regime will change according to their individual health state and their position on their (dynamic) care pathway. On starting dialysis, some medications may be stopped (typically sodium bicarbonate). In the initial few weeks following commencement of dialysis, the patient's antihypertensive medication may also be altered as the patient achieves his or her dry weight (weight without any excess fluid). Patients on haemodialysis may receive some medication in the dialysis unit, e.g. vitamin D or intravenous iron. The type of RRT and the pharmacokinetics of the drug determine the dose of medication required to treat patients with established renal failure on dialysis.

Peritoneal dialysis is a much gentler treatment compared to haemodialysis, Drug removal is by passive diffusion across the peritoneal membrane, so smaller quantities of medication are usually removed.

As haemodialysis is a more aggressive treatment, if a drug is likely to be removed by haemodialysis then it should be given after dialysis. The exception is medication which is given more than three times a day, when it would not be practical to wait until after dialysis to give the drug.

The drugs most likely to be dialysed are those which (Levy *et al.* 2004):

- have a low molecular weight (less than 500 daltons for haemodialysis, up to 30 000 daltons in haemodiafiltration)
- have low protein binding
- have a small volume of distribution (<1 L/kg)
- are highly water-soluble
- are renally excreted (if >50%)

Acute kidney injury

Acute kidney injury (AKI) is defined as a rapid deterioration in renal function, and it can occur over days or weeks. Between 5% and 20% of AKI is drug-related (Ashley 2004), and 2–5% of hospital inpatients will develop AKI, usually due to

Table 8.2 Nephrotoxic drugs.

Diuretics

NSAIDS

ACE inhibitors and ARBs

Calcineurin inhibitors, e.g. ciclosporin, tacrolimus

Radiocontrast media

Beta-blockers

High-dose dopamine

Laxatives

Data from Ashley 2004.

aminoglycosides or radiocontrast media. In primary care ACE inhibitors, ARBs, non-steroidal anti-inflammatory drugs (NSAIDs) and diuretics are the most common causes. As mentioned in Chapter 6, AKI can be subdivided into pre-renal, intra-renal (intrinsic) and post-renal failure, depending on where the injury occurs.

Pre-renal kidney injury

Pre-renal failure is usually due to medication or physiological causes that reduce renal blood flow or cause dehydration. Five per cent of pre-renal failure is due to nephrotoxins. The main drugs implicated are listed in Table 8.2.

Pre-renal kidney injury responds well to the removal of the nephrotoxin and rehydration, and recovery is usually within 24-72 hours once the blood flow is returned to the kidney. If it is not treated quickly enough it can lead to more severe renal impairment, e.g. acute tubular necrosis (ATN). This can happen in primary care mainly in elderly patients who are on an ACE inhibitor and a diuretic and who are unwell and stop eating and drinking for a few days but continue their medication and become dehydrated. When counselling patients on ACE inhibitors or ARBs it is safest to advise them to temporarily discontinue them if they stop drinking for a few days.

Intra-renal kidney injury

Acute damage to the kidney is usually due to a direct nephrotoxic effect on the glomeruli and renal tubules. It can be subdivided into glomerular, hypersensitivity and tubular effects (Table 8.3).

Interstitial nephritis is usually drug-induced, with more than 70 drugs being implicated. Antibiotics, omeprazole and NSAIDs are the most common causes. AKI may occur within two weeks of exposure to the nephrotoxin, or it may be delayed for months. Thirty-five per cent of patients will require dialysis.

ATN is usually due to direct damage to the kidney and causes a reduction in GFR and oliguria or anuria. In some cases it can be prevented by adequate hydration. Contrast-induced nephropathy has an AKI incidence ranging from 0.6% in patients with no renal impairment to 100% in diabetic patients with CKD.

Table 8.3 Nephrotoxic effects of different agents on kidney structure.

Glomerular (immune-mediated)	Hypersensitivity (interstitial nephritis)	Tubular (acute tubular necrosis)
Antibiotics, e.g. penicillin, sulphonamides, rifampicin	Antibiotics, e.g. cephalosporins, erythromycin, penicillin, aminoglycosides, minocycline, rifampicin, sulphonamides	Antibiotics, e.g. aminoglycosides, cephalosporins, colistin, septrin, polymyxin, vancomycin
Allopurinol	Allopurinol	Aciclovir
Halothane	Azathioprine	Amphotericin
NSAIDs	Carbamazepine	Ciclosporin
Gold (2–19% of patients)	Cimetidine	Cisplatin
Penicillamine (30% of patients)	Clofibrate	Lithium
Thiazide diuretics	Diuretics	Heavy metals
	Gold	Herbal medicines
	Halothane	Methyldopa
	Interferon	Mushrooms
	NSAIDs	Paracetamol
	Omeprazole	Radiocontrast media
	Penicillamine	Snake venom
	Phenytoin	

Data from Ashley 2004, Ashley & Morlidge 2008.

Table 8.4 Causes of post-renal kidney injury.

Chemotherapy (due to uric acid crystal formation)

Methysergide (due to retroperitoneal fibrosis)

Sulphonamides

Precipitation of poor-solubility drugs, e.g. intravenous aciclovir, methotrexate

Anticoagulants (due to blood clot formation)

Analgesics

Data from Ashley 2004.

Post-renal kidney injury

This is usually due to obstruction in the urinary tract preventing outflow of urine. It may be caused by disease processes, e.g. malignancy, or due to drugs that cause crystal formation (Table 8.4).

Removal of the obstruction can lead to polyuria, so fluid balance and monitoring of electrolytes is very important to prevent the patient becoming dehydrated, leading to pre-renal kidney injury (see Chapter 6).

Table 8.5 Other drug-related causes of renal impairment.

Vasculitis	Systemic lupus erythematous (SLE)	Rhabdomyolysis
Amphetamines	High-dose hydralazine	Statins
Penicillins	Procainamide	Fibrates
Sulphonamides	Isoniazid	

Data from Ashley 2004.

Table 8.6 Treatment of symptoms in AKI.

Symptom	Treatment
Dehydration	Intravenous/oral fluids
Fluid overload	High-dose diuretics, RRT
Hyperkalaemia	Calcium resonium, glucose/insulin infusions, RRT, dietary potassium restriction
Pulmonary oedema	RRT
Uraemia	RRT
Acidosis	Sodium bicarbonate, RRT
Infection	Treat infections aggressively
Hyperphosphataemia	Dietary phosphate restriction, phosphate binders
Hypocalcaemia	Alfacalcidol and calcium (oral and/or intravenous), but not if the patient has rhabdomyolysis

Other drug-related causes of renal impairment

These are listed in Table 8.5.

Treatment of the symptoms of AKI

The first step is to remove the nephrotoxin, and then the symptoms should be treated (Table 8.6).

Medication used in CKD

Chronic kidney disease mineral and bone disorder (CKD-MBD)

CKD-MBD (or renal osteodystrophy) is caused by the inability of the kidney to regulate phosphate excretion (due to reduced urinary clearance). This leads to reduced calcium absorption and vitamin D metabolism causing stimulation of parathyroid hormone (PTH) production. This results in an increased incidence of fractures and cardiovascular mortality. Almost all patients with CKD stage 4-5 will have some degree of CKD-MBD. The Renal Association standards recommend phosphate levels of 1.1-1.7 mmol/L for dialysis patients and 0.9-1.5 mmol/L for CKD stage 3B-5. This is achieved by a combination of medication (phosphate binders) and diet. Low phosphate levels in haemodialysis patients should be avoided, as they are often an indication of poor nutrition.

There are many different types of phosphate binders available, and the one chosen depends on the patient's blood results (mainly calcium levels) and patient tolerability. Binders work by binding phosphate in the gut and forming a complex with it which is then excreted in the faeces. All phosphate binders should be taken at mealtimes. Patients who are not eating do not need to take any, but if they are having a high-phosphate meal (e.g. macaroni cheese) they should take extra.

The different types of phosphate binders are:

- Calcium-based
  - Calcium carbonate - e.g. Calcichew, Calcium 500
  - Calcium acetate - e.g. Phosex, PhosLo, Renacet, Osvaren (also contains magnesium)
- Heavy-metal-based
  - Aluminium hydroxide - e.g. Alucaps
  - Lanthanum carbonate - e.g Fosrenol
- Polymer-based
  - Sevelamer carbonate and hydrochloride (e.g. Renvela, Renagel)

Alucaps are cheap and effective but they can have quite serious side effects if the aluminium accumulates, which was mainly a problem in the 1960s when dialysis was first introduced. At that time the water used for haemodialysis was not filtered, so if the aluminium content in the water was high this resulted in high aluminium levels in patients, leading to constipation, anaemia, dementia and renal bone disease. They are now only recommended for short-term use.

Calcium-based binders are the main binders used in many units, although they are also losing favour with many nephrologists due to calcium accumulation leading to vascular calcification and cardiovascular mortality. They remain popular as they are inexpensive and are better tolerated than some of the newer phosphate binders such as sevelamer and lanthanum. Calcium acetate is slightly better than calcium carbonate, because less calcium is absorbed. It is important when prescribing calcium carbonate to ensure that it is not the vitamin D formulation (Calcichew D$_3$) that is used, as renal patients are unable to utilise vitamin D in that form. Calcium-based binders should not be taken at the same time as iron tablets, as they form chelates resulting in reduced absorption.

Sevelamer was the first non-calcium, non-aluminium binder licensed. It now comes in two forms as the carbonate (Renvela) and the hydrochloride (Renagel). The tablets are film-coated and easy to swallow, and the carbonate also comes as sachets. They have the advantage that they may slightly lower cholesterol levels. The disadvantages are cost, tablet burden (9-15 tablets have to be taken every day), gastrointestinal side effects and acidosis, and high doses can cause bowel obstruction in peritoneal dialysis patients. They must be taken with or after food; if taken on an empty stomach they are more likely to make the patient feel nauseous.

Lanthanum carbonate is near barium in the periodic table and is visible on abdominal x-rays. The advantages of lanthanum are that it is a non-calcium, non-aluminium binder, it can reduce tablet burden as it comes in different strengths, and it comes as a chewable tablet and granules. It can also be crushed and sprinkled on food. One of the main disadvantages, apart from cost, is its gastrointestinal effects. If taken on an empty stomach it can cause nausea and vomiting.

Vitamin D is essential for healthy bones. The body gets vitamin D from food and the sun in its inactive form (cholecalciferol). In order for it to become useful to the body it must first be metabolised by both the kidney and the liver to active vitamin D (1,25-dihydroxycholecalciferol). In renal failure this process is reduced, which in turn leads to reduced calcium absorption and increased PTH levels.

The calcium range aimed for is the normal range for CKD stage 3-5 and 2.2-2.5 mmol/L for dialysis patients (Renal Association 2010a).

Treatment options are:

- alfacalcidol (1-alpha-hydroxycholecalciferol)
- calcitriol (1,25-dihydroxycholecalciferol)
- vitamin D analogues, e.g. paricalcitol

These can be given either daily or pulsed (three times a week), and by the intravenous or oral route with no difference in efficacy. Haemodialysis patients may receive pulsed therapy in an attempt to minimise the number of tablets they have to take and to ensure adherence. Hypercalcaemia and hyperphosphataemia are the dose-limiting effects. Phosphate should always be corrected before commencing vitamin D. Care should also be taken not to over-suppress the PTH as this can lead to adynamic bone disease. The Renal Association advises aiming for a PTH of 2-9 times the upper limit of normal for the assay used locally.

One of the newest agents used to treat hyperparathyroidsim is cinacalcet, a calcimimetic. It acts on the calcium-sensing receptors on the parathyroid gland and mimics the effects of calcium, reducing PTH secretion. It can produce a reduction in calcium, phosphate, PTH and alkaline phosphatase. Calcium has to be monitored closely initially and after dose changes, as hypocalcaemia can occur. It has been accepted with restrictions by the National Institute for Health and Clinical Excellence (NICE 2007). It is very expensive and is not effective in everyone but can result in savings on erythropoiesis-stimulating agents (ESAs) and phosphate binders and is safer than an operation (parathyroidectomy), which has a high mortality with an average age of 45 years.

Renal anaemia

According to patients, anaemia is one of the most debilitating symptoms of renal disease. It is mainly caused by a lack of erythropoietin production by the kidney, leading to a reduction in red blood cell production by the bone marrow. NICE (2011a) and the Renal Association (2010b) provide guidelines for use in this area.

Renal anaemia can also be caused by:

- iron deficiency
- increased red blood cell breakdown
- blood loss (due to blood tests, haemodialysis or increased GI losses)
- hyperparathyroidism
- aluminium toxicity
- infection or inflammation
- inadequate dialysis

It is best to avoid blood transfusions in patients on the transplant list, to prevent the production of cytotoxic antibodies which can make getting a suitable donor match difficult. Treatment is with a combination of iron and ESAs. NICE and the Renal Association advise starting an ESA if the haemoglobin is below 11 g/dL or if the patient is symptomatic. The ESAs available in the UK are epoetin alfa, beta, theta and zeta, darbepoetin (Aranesp) and methoxy polyethylene glycol-epoetin beta (Mircera). Biosimilars are available for some of the epoetins. It is important to ensure that your patient remains on the same brand and does not switch between them, as they are not interchangeable.

Iron deficiency limits the efficacy of ESA therapy and is the most common cause of non-response to treatment. Patients can be treated with either oral or intravenous iron. Many studies have shown a decrease in ESA maintenance doses with the pre-emptive use of intravenous iron. Intravenous iron is therefore the optimum form in which to give iron to haemodialysis patients and CKD patients on an ESA.

The IV iron products available in the UK are iron sucrose (Venofer), iron dextran (Cosmofer), ferric carboxymaltose (Ferinject) and iron isomaltoside 1000 (Monofer). A test dose is recommended for all intravenous iron preparations apart from Monofer and Ferinject. The main side effects associated with intravenous iron are gastrointestinal upset, injection-site reactions, anaphylactic reactions and hypotension. In practice the main ones are slightly loose stools on the day the patient receives the iron, a metallic taste during the infusion and injection-site reactions. Use intravenous iron with care in people with allergic-type conditions, e.g. asthma and eczema.

The aim of iron treatment is to obtain:

- ferritin 200-500 ng/mL
- transferrin saturation >20%
- hypochromic red cells <6%

The dose of ESA the patient is started on depends on the patient's weight and haemoglobin. Different hospitals have different supply procedures (supplied by the hospital, shared care or home-delivery schemes run by outside companies). The aim of anaemia treatment is to achieve a haemoglobin of 10-12 g/dL with a rise of 1-2 g/dL every month. There have been a number of studies over the past few years that have shown that if you normalise haemoglobin in dialysis patients it can lead to an increase in mortality and vascular access failure (Singh *et al.* 2006, Drueke *et al.* 2006, Renal Association 2010b). Blood pressure (BP) should always be checked prior to administering an ESA injection. Administration should be discussed with medical staff if BP>170/95 mmHg. However, the ESA should not be withheld on the basis of a single BP measurement, but should be discussed with a clinician who will take responsibility for the treatment of the patient's hypertension.

The more common side effects of ESAs are:

- hypertension (usually due to the haemoglobin increasing too quickly)
- flu-like symptoms
- thrombosis
- hyperkalaemia
- seizures

Sodium bicarbonate

This is used to correct the acidosis associated with CKD due to reduced excretion of hydrogen ions by the kidney. If left uncorrected it can lead to respiratory problems and hyperkalaemia. Sodium bicarbonate capsules and tablets are used at doses from 500 mg twice a day, up to 2 g four times a day or more.

Hyperkalaemia

Hyperkalaemia is a common problem in CKD, especially once GFR is below 40–60 mL/min, and it can lead to arrhythmias and death if left untreated. It can be treated with a combination of the following (Levy *et al.* 2004, Ashley 2004):

- removal of potassium-sparing medication, e.g. spironolactone, ACE inhibitors, ARBs, trimethoprim
- dietary potassium (K^+) restriction
- treatment of acidosis – sodium bicarbonate
- 50 mL 50% glucose and short-acting insulin 10 units over 5–10 minutes repeated according to response – lowers K^+ by 1–2 mmol/L over 30–60 minutes
- 10 mL 10% calcium gluconate over 60 seconds to stabilise cardiac muscle
- calcium resonium – works slowly and can cause severe constipation, so always prescribe with a laxative
- salbutamol nebules (lowers K^+ by 0.6–1 mmol/L)
- dialysis

Hypertension

Hypertension can be both cause and effect of renal impairment, and it affects approximately 80–90% of renal patients. It is defined as BP ≥140/90 mmHg measured on three separate occasions. Malignant hypertension, defined as

BP >180/110 mmHg with progressive organ damage and papilloedema, must be treated immediately. Guidelines from NICE (2011b) and the Renal Association (2011) are available on the treatment of hypertension.

BP aimed for:

- with proteinuria >1 g/24 h or diabetic
  - Renal Association: <130/80 mmHg
- without proteinuria
  - NICE: <140/90 mmHg
  - Renal Association: <140/90 mmHg

The latest update to NICE (2011b) aims for a BP target of <150/90 mmHg in patients over 80 years of age.

Renal hypertension is mainly due to increased activity of the renin-angiotensin system (RAS) causing sodium and water retention. It must be adequately controlled to limit the rate of decline of kidney function and decrease the risk of cardiovascular mortality. Rarely is it controlled by one drug, and a combination is usually required.

Drug therapies available:

- beta-adrenoceptor blocking drugs
- calcium-channel blockers
- drugs affecting the RAS
- alpha-adrenoceptor blocking drugs
- centrally acting agents
- diuretics

Beta-adrenoceptor blocking drugs

According to NICE (2011b), these should be used in younger patients who are intolerant of ACE inhibitors or ARBs. In renal patients beta-blockade is best achieved with bisoprolol, carvedilol or metoprolol as they are dual or hepatically excreted. In practice most are well tolerated, but always start with a low dose and gradually increase the dose as tolerated. Beta-blockers are best avoided if clinically possible in people with new fistulas as they can decrease the blood flow to the fistula and cause maturation problems. Water-soluble beta-blockers are less likely to cause sleep disturbances but are usually renally excreted, and therefore may accumulate in renal failure – although this is not usually a problem.

Calcium-channel blockers

These are first-line agents in patients >55 years old and in black African or Caribbean patients (NICE 2011b). One limitation is ankle swelling; this is more frequent with the dihydropyridines such as amlodipine. Diltiazem is sometimes used to reduce proteinuria. Lercanidipine, nicardipine, diltiazem and verapamil may cause an increase in ciclosporin levels, so they should be used with care in transplant patients. Verapamil can also cause constipation.

Drugs affecting the RAS

These are first-line agents for patients <55 years old and can be subdivided into ACE inhibitors, ARBs and renin inhibitors (e.g. aliskiren) (NICE 2011b). They have cardio- and reno-protective effects. ARBs are less likely to cause the cough associated with ACE inhibitors, because they do not affect bradykinin. ACE inhibitors and ARBs are two of the main treatments for diabetic nephropathy and proteinuria as they can prevent the rate of decline of renal function. They exert their reno-protective effect by reducing proteinuria, increasing GFR and reducing arterial blood pressure. They should be used with caution in patients with renal artery stenosis or dehydration, where they may cause a reduction in GFR. When initiating treatment, especially in haemodialysis patients, start with a small dose at night. Hyperkalaemia and increased creatinine are the dose-limiting factors associated with this class of antihypertensive. An increase in creatinine of 20% should be expected. Urea and electrolytes (U&Es) should be monitored every 1–2 weeks after starting and dose alterations.

Alpha-adrenoceptor blocking drugs

Alpha-blockers are not first-line agents but are used in conjunction with other antihypertensives, as renal patients usually have resistant hypertension. They also have the advantage that they can lower cholesterol levels and help with urinary retention in benign prostatic hyperplasia.

Centrally acting agents

As renal hypertension is so difficult to treat, centrally acting agents may also be used, e.g. moxonidine or methyldopa, but side effects such as tiredness tend to limit the long-term use of the latter. Vasodilatory agents, e.g. hydralazine or minoxidil, are other alternatives, although side effects such as hirsutism may limit the use of minoxidil, and fluid retention and systemic lupus erythematosis (in high doses) that of hydralazine.

Diuretics

Thiazide diuretics such as bendroflumethiazide are ineffective if creatinine clearance is less than 30 mL/min. Metolazone has a role in combination with loop diuretics to help remove fluid in resistant oedema. Metolazone is now unlicensed but can be imported from IDIS.

   Loop diuretics – A normal dose of furosemide in CKD can be from 250 mg to 2 g per day. If the oral formulation does not work then intravenous furosemide is indicated, but monitor for signs of deafness, which are usually reversible. Bumetanide can also be used and may be beneficial in patients in whom furosemide is not working. A rough conversion is 1 mg of bumetanide = 40 mg of furosemide.

   Prolonged diuretic therapy can also lead to fluid depletion, which can cause AKI, so check the patient's weight before and during therapy. Monitoring a patient's weight is the best way to assess fluid balance, as urine collections are notoriously inaccurate.

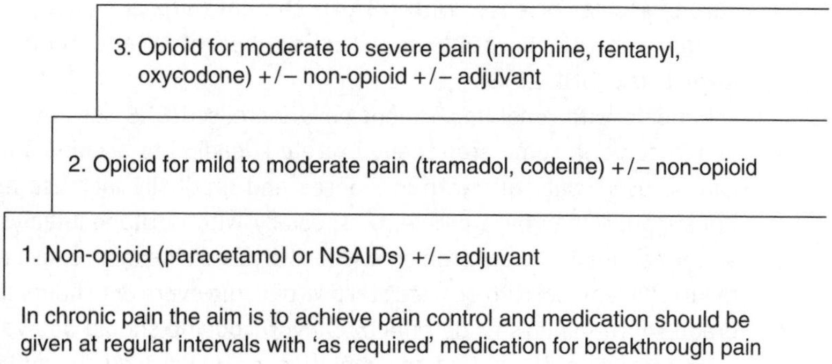

3. Opioid for moderate to severe pain (morphine, fentanyl, oxycodone) +/− non-opioid +/− adjuvant

2. Opioid for mild to moderate pain (tramadol, codeine) +/− non-opioid

1. Non-opioid (paracetamol or NSAIDs) +/− adjuvant

In chronic pain the aim is to achieve pain control and medication should be given at regular intervals with 'as required' medication for breakthrough pain

Figure 8.1 Analgesic ladder for chronic pain.

With haemodialysis, urine output tails off the longer the patient is on haemodialysis, so diuretics would be ineffective in treating oedema and fluid-related hypertension. In this case adjustment to the patient's dry weight can be instituted.

Analgesia

Pain is a very difficult symptom to control in renal impairment, and it can be due to a variety of causes, including dialysis-related headaches, arthritis, phantom limb pain, cancer, to name but a few. As for all patients with chronic pain, the analgesic ladder (Figure 8.1) should be followed.

Paracetamol is the main drug for mild to moderate pain in renal patients, and no dose reduction is required for oral treatment, although for intravenous administration the frequency should be no more than every six to eight hours.

Non-steroidal anti-inflammatory drugs (NSAIDs) affect renal prostaglandins and are contraindicated in CKD patients not on dialysis as they reduce GFR. In dialysis patients NSAIDs can be prescribed if the patient is anuric – but use with caution if a patient on dialysis passes urine. It is important to remember that many patients on dialysis retain some function, and a useful urine output allows them more freedom in terms of fluid intake and a reduction in the number of hours on dialysis or peritoneal dialysis exchanges. This may be lost if an NSAID is prescribed. Loss of residual renal function in peritoneal dialysis patients may critically reduce weekly clearance of creatinine such that patients require to convert to haemodialysis.

Dialysis patients are at an increased risk of gastrointestinal side effects, so always ensure that they receive stomach protection for the duration of the course. Although Cox-IIs are thought to have less effect on renal prostaglandins, they should also be avoided in patients with CKD who are not on dialysis, similarly to the NSAIDs. Cox-IIs and COX-II selective NSAIDs are associated with an increased risk of thrombotic events (e.g. myocardial infarction and stroke), so if at all possible they should be avoided in patients with renal disease, who already have an increased risk of cardiovascular disease. With NSAIDs the data are less clear; diclofenac is associated with the greatest risk, then ibuprofen, and naproxen has the lowest risk (BNF 2012).

Patients with renal impairment have increased CNS sensitivity to opioids, and in addition some are renally excreted, leading to accumulation. Codeine can be used, but start with low doses and gradually increase as tolerated. Constipation may be a problem, especially with peritoneal dialysis patients, and it can lead to flow problems with dialysis exchanges, causing treatment failure. If tramadol is to be used start with 50 mg every 8–12 hours and increase gradually to minimise side effects. Dihydrocodeine should be avoided if possible because of the risk of accumulation, as dihydrocodeine and its metabolites are renally excreted.

Patients with CKD stages 3–5 requiring strong opioid analgesia are best treated with 2.5–5 mg of morphine no more than eight-hourly initially. The metabolites of morphine (morphine-6-glucuronide, a renally excreted active metabolite more potent than morphine, and morphine-3-glucuronide) can accumulate, resulting in an increased effect. The half-life of morphine-6-glucuronide is increased from 3–5 hours in normal renal function to 50 hours in CKD 5. Patients should be observed carefully for signs of accumulation. Sustained-release preparations such as MST or Zomorph should be used with great care, as accumulation may take a few days – so it is very important to gradually titrate doses. Oxycodone should be treated like morphine – i.e. start with a small dose and gradually titrate upwards. Although it is sometimes slightly better tolerated than morphine by renal patients, the same problems with accumulation are seen. Patches of fentanyl and buprenorphine can also be used. Again, low doses are recommended – e.g. start with fentanyl 12 μg every three days and with the lowest buprenorphine patch. Pethidine does have a role in renal colic but should otherwise be avoided because of the risk of accumulation. The Liverpool Care Pathway for end-of-life care recommends using fentanyl or alfentanil as first line, with oxycodone and morphine being alternatives if they are unavailable. Fentanyl and alfentanil have the advantage that they are hepatically metabolised, so less accumulation should occur.

Adjuvants are drugs not normally classified as analgesics but which can be used for neuropathic or phantom limb pain (e.g. anticonvulsants, antidepressants). It is very important when commencing these therapies in people with renal impairment that a very low dose is used initially to minimise any side effects – e.g. amitriptyline 25 mg at night, gabapentin 100 mg daily and pregabalin 25 mg daily. The dose can then slowly be increased in 1–2 weekly intervals depending on patient tolerability. If it is increased too quickly it can result in nausea, drowsiness, confusion and a fear of using the drug.

Remember that patients should always be treated as individuals. Each patient can tolerate different amounts of analgesia. The 80-year-old 50 kg woman has been known to tolerate larger doses of analgesia than the 40-year-old 100 kg man!

Hepatitis B vaccine

Vaccination of all patients and staff entering a renal unit is desirable, to protect both patients and staff from infection. This has been known to be a hazard since the 1960s. Although it is now very rare, there was an outbreak in Edinburgh in 1969/70 in which 40 members of staff and patients were infected, and seven patients and four members of staff died.

All patients have their immune status checked before commencing haemodialysis. Renal patients are immunocompromised and do not respond as well to the vaccine, and therefore require a more intensive course. Response is greater if vaccination is commenced before dialysis is required. Patients usually receive three or four doses of 40 µg, and depending on what make of vaccine is administered a repeat course may be necessary. The aim is to achieve a titre >10 mIU/mL.

Antibiotics and antiviral agents

Many antibiotics and antiviral agents are renally excreted, so care should be taken with dosing. Doses should be adjusted depending on the clinical situation and response of the patient. Most penicillins and cephalosporins can be given at normal doses, although care should be exercised at maximum doses. Exceptions are benzylpenicillin and ceftazidime, both of which are very neurotoxic and should be given in greatly reduced doses.

Nitrofurantoin should be avoided, because in order to work it has to concentrate in the urine – and therefore in patients who pass no or very little urine it is unlikely to be effective.

Tetracyclines should be used with care, although doxycycline can safely be given at normal doses in all stages of renal impairment.

Macrolides, e.g. erythromycin and clarithromycin, and quinolones, e.g. ciprofloxacin, can cause nausea if used in high doses. Normal doses can be used for clarithromycin and ciprofloxacin for short courses, but if the course is extended, e.g. for endocarditis, the dose may require to be reduced to limit side effects. The maximum recommended dose of erythromycin is 2 g daily.

Drugs such as gentamicin and vancomycin should be used at greatly reduced doses and frequencies, and dosed according to levels.

At least 50% of aminoglycosides are dialysed out, so for haemodialysis patients it is important to know when the level was taken in order to determine the appropriate dose.

When using vancomycin in haemodialysis patients, a single dose of 1 g should be given intravenously over 100 minutes and trough levels monitored. The next dose would then be given when the trough level falls to 10-15 mg/L (15-20 mg/L in some protocols). A single dose will often last between two and seven days depending on urine output and mode of dialysis. More vancomycin is removed by haemodiafiltration (HDF) than by haemodialysis, so post-dialysis dosing is usually required for HDF.

Clostridium difficile is a major problem in the renal population, as these patients are immunocompromised and can receive frequent courses of antibiotics. Metronidazole should be used first line, but in recurrent cases oral vancomycin should be prescribed. A new agent called fidaxomicin was licensed in 2012, and in trials this has been shown to be superior to vancomycin.

Antiviral agents accumulate in renal failure and cause neurotoxicity, so a markedly reduced dose should be used. For example, for herpes zoster, aciclovir 400-800 mg twice daily should be used. Contact the renal unit or renal pharmacist for advice on dosing.

Timing of medication administration in haemodialysis patients is also important, especially for once-daily dosing, where patients should be advised to take their medication after dialysis. Some medication is also recommended to be taken with large quantities of water, which again is not always possible for renal patients, and they should be advised to remain within their fluid restriction.

Dialysis-related conditions

Haemodialysis patients commonly complain of cramp, either during haemodialysis due to rapid electrolyte or fluid shifts, or at night. Quinine sulphate 200 mg daily is the drug of choice.

Restless legs (the involuntary jerking of limbs) is another common complaint, and this can lead to sleepless nights for both the patient and his or her partner. It can be treated with a variety of drugs, the most commonly used being the drugs used for Parkinson's disease such as Madopar (unlicensed use), ropinirole or pramipexole. These are started with a low daily dose and gradually increased according to response. Previously clonazepam 0.5-4 mg at night was the drug of choice, although drowsiness can be a problem at higher doses. Because of the addiction potential of benzodiazepines, the Parkinson's drugs are now tried first, although clonazepam remains the most effective treatment. Buprenorphine patches have also been used. Tolerance may develop to the medication used to treat restless legs, so patients may rotate through a few different treatments, and sometimes a drug holiday can be beneficial.

Concordance

Concordance should be distinguished from compliance. Compliance is part of a paternalistic approach to patient care, where patients are expected to comply with what healthcare professionals tell them to do. Concordance (or adherence) implies a joint, non-judgemental approach to treatment where all the options are outlined to the patient and a partnership is formed with the health professional.

Concordance in patients with long-term conditions is extremely problematic and can relate to medication, diet or dialysis. Studies show that up to 30% of

Table 8.7 Causes of 'unintentional' and 'intentional' non-adherence (Pruce 2011), and possible solutions.

Unintentional		Intentional	
Causes	Solutions	Causes	Solutions
Forgetfulness (may be related to stress, alcohol, age etc.)	Reminders, e.g. alarms, text messaging	Fears, e.g. side effects, dependence	Education
Confusion	Charts and/or record sheets	Lack of trust	Motivational counselling
Not in a routine	Compliance boxes		Psychologists
Complicated regime	Simplify regime, use combination preparations		Communication
			Empowerment
Unable to use inhaler, open bottle	Aids, e.g. Haleraid, Volumatic, non-child-resistant caps		

patients are not taking their medication at any one time. This leads to a major waste of resources for the National Health Service (NHS). Studies in transplant patients put this at 16–55%, and it can result in organ rejection and loss of the transplanted kidney (Wells 2004).

Non-adherence can vary within individuals over time. It is most common in patients who are:

- younger
- male
- smokers
- poorly educated
- single
- depressed
- low income
- lacking in support
- suffering from comorbidities
- taking several medications (renal patients may be taking 10–20 different drugs)

It was thought that improving patient knowledge of their medication would improve adherence, but studies are divided in their outcomes. Patient education should still be promoted, as there is a link between understanding, memory, satisfaction and compliance. When counselling patients, it is very important to be non-judgemental.

Some authors have divided non-adherence into unintentional and intentional, depending on the cause (Pruce 2011). Reasons for non-adherence, and possible solutions, are listed in Table 8.7.

Transplantation and immunosuppression

Transplantation has the best life expectancy and is the most cost-effective method of RRT. There are many different medication regimes used for transplantation. Factors that influence the combination used include:

- degree of donor match
- living or cadaveric donor
- transplant history
- ethnicity
- concomitant conditions, e.g. HIV, diabetes.
- patient preference with respect to side effects of medication

The aim of transplant medication is to maximise graft survival with minimal adverse effects, e.g. malignancy, infection and cardiovascular disease. NICE (2004) has issued guidelines on which medication should be used, with alternative options for specific situations.

Triple therapy using drugs with differing mechanisms of action is the most common regimen. When patients are first transplanted they are on higher doses of medication, and higher drug levels are needed. After a few months, as long as there have been no problems with rejection, then the doses can be titrated down. Live vaccines should not be given to transplant patients.

The main classes of immunosuppressants are:

- calcineurin inhibitors (e.g. tacrolimus, ciclosporin)
- antiproliferative agents (e.g. azathioprine, mycophenolate)
- corticosteroids (e.g. prednisolone)
- mTOR inhibitors (e.g. sirolimus)
- monoclonal antibodies (e.g. ATG, basiliximab, alemtuzumab)

Calcineurin inhibitors (CNIs)

These drugs inhibit interleukin 2 (IL-2) transcription and decrease T-cell proliferation. Examples include tacrolimus and ciclosporin. General side effects include:

- nephrotoxicity
- hypertension
- hyperkalaemia
- hyperlipidaemia

Ciclosporin can also cause gingival hyperplasia, acne, hirsutism, hypertrichosis, gastrointestinal effects, diabetes and myalgia. Tacrolimus can also cause diabetes, alopecia and neurotoxicity, e.g. tremor, headache. Tacrolimus is now the preferred agent, as it has been shown to have fewer episodes of rejection and improved graft survival.

Calcineurin inhibitors are metabolised by the CYP450 3A4 system and therefore have numerous drug interactions. The most common drug interactions are with antibiotics, antivirals, antifungals, antihypertensives, anticonvulsants, calcium-channel blockers, warfarin and lipid-lowering medication. If patients are started or discontinued on an interacting medication, ensure that levels are checked within a few days. Levels are taken immediately pre-dose.

Since CNIs are dosed according to levels it is very important that the patient always receives the same brand of medication.

Ciclosporin comes in two forms: Sandimmun (which is only available on a named patient basis) and Neoral. They have different dosage frequencies; the most common form is Neoral.

Tacrolimus also comes in two forms: immediate-release (Prograf) and prolonged-release (Advagraf), which have different frequencies of administration and are not interchangeable.

A number of branded generic formulations of the immediate-release preparation are now available (Adoport, Vivadex, Tacni). It is very important that the patient remains on the brand prescribed by the transplant unit. Differences in bioavailability between brands can result in fluctuations in tacrolimus or ciclosporin levels, leading to increased toxicity or graft loss.

CNIs should always be prescribed by brand rather than generically, to prevent confusion.

Antiproliferative agents

These are used in combination with calcineurin inhibitors. Examples are azathioprine and mycophenolate.

Azathioprine
Azathioprine is metabolised to 6-mercaptopurine. It interferes with DNA and RNA synthesis, leading to a reduction of activated B and T cells. The main side effects are:

- myelosuppression
- increased sensitivity to infections
- hypersensitivity reactions
- alopecia
- nausea

It should never be given with allopurinol, which can reduce the metabolism of azathioprine and result in severe haematological toxicity.

Mycophenolate
Mycophenolate mofetil (MMF) is metabolised to the active form mycophenolic acid (MPA). MPA interferes with purine biosynthesis, which in turn inhibits

DNA synthesis and therefore prevents B-cell and T-cell proliferation. Side effects include:

- increased sensitivity to infections, especially viral
- gastrointestinal effects, usually nausea, vomiting or diarrhoea (if patients are having problems tolerating them then the dose may be reduced and/or the frequency increased)
- myelosuppression, especially leucopenia and anaemia

Mycophenolate comes in two forms: as the mofetil salt (CellCept) and as mycophenolate sodium (Myfortic), and again the two have completely different doses and cannot be interchanged. Generic substitution of mycophenolate mofetil is possible, as it is not blood-level-dependent. The MHRA has issued advice to say that all generic brands of MMF are interchangeable with CellCept.

Corticosteroids

Examples include methylprednisolone and prednisolone (Popat 2010). Methylprednisolone is usually used either for induction or for treatment of acute rejection. Prednisolone is used for maintenance therapy in combination with a CNI and an antiproliferative agent.

The mechanism of action is not completely understood. they prevent T-cell activation and the production of macrophage cytokines (e.g. interleukins, interferons and tumour necrosis factors). Side effects include (BNF 2012):

- sodium and water retention
- Cushing's syndrome
- GI toxicity
- weight gain
- skin thinning
- osteoporosis
- diabetes

The dose is usually reduced to as low a dose as possible or even stopped once the patient is 6-12 months post transplant.

It is best to use uncoated prednisolone, especially with high doses, to ensure that the patient is receiving the correct dose (enteric-coated formulations have an unpredictable absorption profile).

mTOR inhibitors

This class of drugs includes sirolimus (Ashley 2010, Popat 2010). They inhibit T-cell, B-cell and vascular smooth muscle proliferation by blocking intracellular signal transduction. Side effects include:

- delayed wound healing
- hyperlipidaemia

- thrombocytopenia
- mouth ulcers
- pneumonitis
- arthralgia
- peripheral oedema

The main advantage with sirolimus is lack of nephrotoxicity, and therefore it can be used in place of the CNIs. NICE (2004) advocates using it only in proven CNI intolerance. Blood levels are monitored to minimise toxicity. It should not be given at the same time as ciclosporin, as ciclosporin can increase sirolimus levels. Sirolimus is also metabolised by the CYP450 3A4 system, so it has a number of interactions mainly with antibacterials, antifungals, antivirals, calcium-channel blockers and grapefruit juice (BNF 2012).

Polyclonal and monoclonal antibodies

Examples are anti-thymocyte immunoglobulin (rabbit) (ATG), basiliximab, alemtuzumab, rituximab. These drugs are only used in transplant centres under specialist supervision. They are used as induction to reduce the risk of acute rejection and delayed graft function, and for the treatment of acute rejection. If the kidney is a very good match, e.g. a kidney from a twin, then induction therapy may not be required, but it is given in the majority of cases.

Complications

The complications of immunosuppression include cardiovascular disease, increased risk of infections and cancer. Malignancy is 3–5 times more common in transplant patients, so they are closely monitored at transplant clinics. Urinary tract infections are common and need treatment with a slightly extended antibiotic course.

A number of different medications are given to prevent some of the infections and complications associated with immunosuppression (Ashley & Morlidge 2008, Ashley 2010):

- Co-trimoxazole 480–960 mg daily for the first few months to prevent *Pneumocystis jirovecii* (*P. carinii*) pneumonia.
- Aciclovir, ganciclovir or valganciclovir for the first three months to prevent cytomegalovirus (CMV). Those most at risk are CMV-negative recipients who receive a CMV-positive kidney.
- Nystatin to prevent candida.
- Isoniazid 200–300 mg daily for 6–12 months to prevent tuberculosis (TB) in high-risk patients, e.g. black African and South-East Asian patients or patients with a history of previous TB.
- Proton-pump inhibitors (e.g. omeprazole, lansoprazole) or H_2 antagonists (e.g. ranitidine) to prevent peptic ulcers.
- Bisphosphonates to prevent corticosteroid-induced osteoporosis.

- Hypertension and hyperlipidaemia should be treated to minimise cardiovascular complications.
- Aspirin to prevent clot formation in the renal transplant vasculature.

Over-the-counter and complementary therapies

Care should be taken when advising on over-the-counter (OTC) medication or complementary therapies for renal patients, because of interactions with their prescribed medication, altered pharmacokinetics in CKD or nephrotoxicity.

Some medication to take particular care with is:

- cod liver oil capsules
- cough and cold remedies
- indigestion and wind remedies
- herbal medicines
- painkillers except paracetamol

Cod liver oil preparations may contain calcium, iron, and vitamins A, B, C and D. Vitamin D is usually in a form which cannot be utilised by people with CKD. Vitamin A can cause abnormal calcium metabolism and is renally excreted, so toxic levels may occur.

Fish oils are sometimes recommended for certain groups of patients, but all contraindications should first be assessed. High doses of fish oils may also reduce the immune system so should not be used in immunosuppressed patients and those with various comorbidities. Omega-3 fatty acids may have a role in the treatment of IgA nephropathy.

Cough and cold remedies may contain ingredients which can increase blood pressure, e.g. pseudoephedrine found in Actifed, Sudafed and Benylin to name a few. They may also contain vitamin C, which can cause kidney stones, or paracetamol, which could lead to an inadvertent overdose, e.g. Day Nurse. For coughs and colds the safest things to advise patients to take are:

- for congestion: menthol inhalations or Karvol capsules
- for a sore throat: simple linctus or buttercup syrup
- for a cough: pholcodine linctus
- for flu-like symptoms: paracetamol and a hot drink

Take care with diabetic patients, as they should receive sugar-free preparations.

Indigestion and wind remedies, e.g. Rennies, usually contain calcium carbonate. This may be in the patient's prescribed phosphate binder and if taken outside of meal times may lead to high calcium levels. Other indigestion remedies may contain aluminium, which can accumulate in renal impairment and lead to the problems described earlier. The best option is to start stomach protection, e.g. H_2-antagonists or proton-pump inhibitors (PPIs), or advise the patient to take Gaviscon / Peptac or peppermint water. Care should be taken with omeprazole because of its interaction with clopidogrel, which may cause a reduced antiplatelet effect and increase the risk of atherothrombotic events in high-risk patients. PPIs have also been implicated in the increased incidence of *Clostridium difficile* infections.

Complementary therapies are increasing in popularity as people are becoming disillusioned by conventional medicine (which they see as impersonal) and the related side effects. Renal patients are no different to anyone else – they want something that will cure their dialysis-related symptoms without causing side effects.

The majority of homeopathic medication is safe to use, but again it should be assessed in each individual case. Herbal remedies can cause more problems, because:

- Many are unlicensed, so they can vary greatly in toxicity and purity, due to differences in harvesting or environmental factors.
- They may contain contaminants.
- They may interact with prescribed medication.
- They may be nephrotoxic or hepatotoxic.

It is hoped, however, that with the EU Directive governing the safety and quality of herbal medication (Directive 2004/24/EC) coming into force in May 2011, some of these problems may be resolved.

Conclusion

Renal patients are a diverse group, and medication should be dosed accordingly. CKD is very common in the elderly population, and dosage adjustments should always be considered when prescribing for them. Every patient should be treated as an individual. Promotion of continuity and consistency of care for patients with kidney disease is facilitated through collaborative links with specialist services. Renal units are important as a useful resource in managing patients with CKD, and staff are more than happy to offer prescribing advice or support in managing recalcitrant symptoms.

References and resources

Aronoff, G.R., Bennett, W.M., Berns, J.S, *et al*. (2007) *Drug Prescribing in Renal Failure: Dosing Guidelines for Adults*, 5th edition. American College of Physicians, Philadelphia.

Ashley, C. (2004) Renal failure: how drugs can damage the kidney. *Hospital Pharmacist*, **11**, 48–53.

Ashley, C. & Morlidge C. (2008) *Introduction to Renal Therapeutics*. Pharmaceutical Press, London.

Ashley, C. & Currie A. (2009) *The Renal Drug Handbook*, 3rd edition. Radcliffe Medical Press, Oxford.

Ashley C. (2010) Challenges of transplantation: what are the drug options? *British Journal of Clinical Pharmacy*, **2**, 77–83.

BNF (2012) *British National Formulary 63*. British Medical Association and Royal Pharmaceutical Society of Great Britain, London.

Daugirdas, J.T., Blake, P.G. & Ing, T.S. (2007) *Handbook of Dialysis*, 4th edition. Lippincott Williams & Wilkins, Philadelphia.

Devaney, A., Ashley, C. & Tomson, C. (2006) How the reclassification of kidney disease impacts on dosage adjustments. *Pharmaceutical Journal*, **277**, 403-4.

Drueke, T.B., Locatelli, F., Clyne, N. *et al.*; CREATE Investigators (2006) Normalization of hemoglobin level in patients with chronic kidney disease and anemia. *New England Journal of Medicine*, **355**, 2071–84.

Levy, J., Morgan, J., Brown, E. (2004) *Oxford Handbook of Dialysis*, 2nd edition. Oxford University Press, Oxford.

Liverpool Care Pathway for the Dying Patient (LCP). http://www.mcpcil.org.uk (accessed September 2012).

NICE (2004) *Renal transplantation: immunosuppressive regimens (adults)*. Technology Appraisal 85. National Institute for Health and Clinical Excellence, London. http://www.nice.org.uk/TA85 (accessed September 2012).

NICE (2007) *Cinacalcet for the treatment of secondary hyperparathyroidism in patients with end-stage renal disease on maintenance dialysis therapy*. Technology Appraisal 117. National Institute for Health and Clinical Excellence, London. http://www.nice.org.uk/TA117 (accessed September 2012).

NICE (2011a) *Anaemia management in people with chronic kidney disease*. Clinical Guideline 114. National Institute for Health and Clinical Excellence, London. http://www.nice.org.uk/CG114 (accessed September 2012).

NICE (2011b) *Hypertension: clinical management of primary hypertension in adults*. Clinical Guideline 127. National Institute for Health and Clinical Excellence, London. http://www.nice.org.uk/CG127 (accessed September 2012).

Popat, R. (2010) Organ transplantation: immunosuppression. *Clinical Pharmacist*, **2**, 48-52.

Pruce, D. (2011) Addressing poor medication adherence. *Pharmaceutical Journal*, **286**, 172.

Renal Association (2009) Clinical practice guidelines: blood borne virus infection. http://www.renal.org/Clinical/GuidelinesSection/Guidelines.aspx (accessed September 2012).

Renal Association (2010a) Clinical practice guidelines: CKD-mineral and bone diseases, 5th edition. http://www.renal.org/Clinical/GuidelinesSection/Guidelines.aspx (accessed September 2012).

Renal Association (2010b) Clinical practice guidelines: anaemia of CKD, 5th edition. http://www.renal.org/Clinical/GuidelinesSection/Guidelines.aspx (accessed September 2012).

Renal Association (2011) Detection, monitoring and care of patients with CKD. http://www.renal.org/Clinical/GuidelinesSection/Guidelines.aspx (accessed September 2012).

Singh, A.K., Szczech, L., Tang, K.L. *et al.*; CHOIR Investigators (2006) Correction of anemia with epoetin alfa in chronic kidney disease. *New England Journal of Medicine*, **355**, 2085-98.

Spruill, W.J., Wade, W.E. & Cobb, H.H. (2007) Estimating glomerular filtration rate with a modification of diet in renal disease equation: implications for pharmacy. *American Journal of Health-System Pharmacy*, **64**, 652-60.

Wells, H. (2004) Promoting adherence in renal transplant patients. *Hospital Pharmacist*, **11**, 69-71.

Chapter 9
Optimising Nutrition in People with Chronic Kidney Disease

Helena Jackson[1] and Sally Noble[2]

[1]Renal Dietitian, St George's Hospital, London, UK
[2]Renal Dietitian, Logan Hospital, Brisbane, Australia

Introduction

This chapter aims to describe the main aspects of diet in chronic kidney disease (CKD) and to provide non-specialists with practical information on managing the dietary requirements of patients on renal replacement therapy (RRT) and post renal transplant. There is no single diet for people with kidney disease, but most people will need to adapt their diet according to the stage and effects of their condition. The diet also needs to be individualised for each patient according to factors such as socioeconomic background, religious and pre-existing dietary restrictions and other clinical conditions.

Dietary treatment can be grouped broadly into three main areas:

(1) maintaining a healthy, balanced diet in terms of macro- and micronutrient intakes and chronic disease prevention
(2) control of waste products and toxins, which is a function of healthy kidneys
(3) prevention and treatment of malnutrition

Patients with advanced disease will often be well versed in their dietary regimes, and in the first instance non-specialists can often establish important dietary principles from the patient and or their family. Where more detailed information is needed or the patient requires a specialist review, renal dietitians are easily accessible through the patient's kidney unit.

Kidney Disease Management: A Practical Approach for the Non-Specialist Healthcare Practitioner, First Edition. Edited by Rachel Lewis and Helen Noble.
© 2013 John Wiley & Sons, Ltd. Published 2013 by John Wiley & Sons, Ltd.

Specialist dietitians

Individuals on dialysis or receiving a transplant will have renal dietitians assigned to their unit and should be seen promptly for dietetic treatment, with regular follow-up and review. Other outpatients with CKD stages 3–5 may have access to a renal dietitian at nephrology clinic, diabetes clinic or other specialist centre. However, many patients would welcome dietary advice at an earlier stage. The experienced clinician can safely and effectively provide initial advice, for example on healthy eating, low-salt and low-potassium diets (see Figure 9.2). However, a referral to a dietitian can be helpful if outcomes are not being achieved.

CKD patients who would benefit from a renal dietetic referral include:

- Patients with CKD stage 5, particularly those new to peritoneal dialysis or haemodialysis, and those choosing conservative management.
- Patients with CKD stage 4–5, with reduced appetite or intake, or any symptoms such as nausea or dysphagia that may compromise intake, as well as those with actual weight loss.
- CKD patients with chronic conditions such as cancer and gastrointestinal disorders that increase the risk of malnutrition.
- Patients following multiple dietary restrictions such as vegan, low-potassium and/or low-phosphate diets.
- Those following a low-phosphate diet and needing advice on the use of phosphate binders in relation to intake (some renal dietitians are prescribers of phosphate binders).

CKD and healthy eating

Prevention

Diet has an important role in reducing the risk of developing CKD and delaying its progression. This is primarily due to the contribution of diet to the management of chronic conditions such as hypertension, diabetes and obesity.

Healthy eating guidelines for CKD

In patients with existing CKD, diet and lifestyle remain important modifiable risk factors. National healthy eating guidelines are applicable in most cases and can be adapted for dialysis patients and others on restrictive therapeutic diets. There are specific guidelines for the role of diet in managing chronic conditions in patients with CKD (KDOQI 2007). UK national guidelines emphasise the need for a balance between energy needs and nutrient requirements so that energy intake should not exceed or fall short of requirements. People with CKD have similar energy requirements to the general population, but those on dialysis are at an increased risk of an energy deficit, and the guidelines reflect this (Ash et al. 2006).

General recommendations suggest eating a wide range of foods for a balanced intake of nutrients. This applies equally to patients with CKD on restricted diets. If this cannot be achieved they should be referred to a dietitian. Particular caution should be exercised with certain dietary approaches that result in an imbalance of particular nutrients such as:

- high-protein, low-carbohydrate diets
- very high intake of fruit or vegetables (risk of high serum potassium levels)
- high intake of dairy products (risk of excess phosphate/protein/potassium intake)

The healthy eating guidelines are summarised below, with comments on their applicability to individuals with CKD.

- **Base meals on starchy foods** (potatoes, cereals, pasta, rice and bread) – Where possible, wholegrain varieties and unsalted options should be chosen. Starchy foods should amount to a third of total food intake. People on a low-potassium diet will need to boil potatoes, yams and other starchy vegetables before eating or cooking further.
- **Eat lots of fruit and vegetables** - Five (80 g) portions of different types of fruit and vegetables a day are recommended. Even on a low-potassium diet one should maintain total fruit and vegetable intake as much as possible, and most patients can include at least four daily portions with the correct advice (see section on potassium, below).
- **Eat more fish** – At least two portions a week should be eaten, including one portion of oily fish. If possible, fish should be fresh, frozen or canned in spring water, as alternatives can be high in salt. Oily fish is high in omega-3 fats, which may help to prevent heart disease. Low-phosphate diets usually limit oily fish to no more than once or twice weekly and restrict fish with edible bones such as whitebait and tinned fish.
- **Cut down on saturated fat and sugar** – Saturated fat is associated with an increased risk of high cholesterol levels and cardiovascular disease. It is found in butter, lard, meat fat, cream, hard cheese, sausages, pies and many cakes and biscuits. Unsaturated vegetable oils and margarines are preferable. All fats have a high energy content, and limiting intakes will help to reduce the risk of becoming overweight. Sugary foods and drinks are often high in calories and low in other nutrients. However, In patients with poor appetites and an energy deficit, increasing dietary fat and sugar can be a practical and palatable way to optimise energy intake.
- **Eat less salt** – Eating less salt can reduce the risk of CKD, hypertension, stroke and heart disease in the general population and the progression in existing CKD. In more advanced CKD, a lower salt intake will help reduce the risk of fluid retention and is generally essential for patients requiring a fluid restriction.

- **Get active and be a healthy weight** – Overweight and obesity increase the risk of hypertension, diabetes, cardiovascular disease and CKD in the general population and are associated with more rapid progression in established CKD. Transplant candidates usually need to have a body mass index (BMI) below a maximum upper limit, typically 30–35 kg/m^2, and aim for a healthy weight (BMI 20–25 kg/m^2) post transplant. However, in dialysis patients there is evidence that heavier individuals have a lower mortality risk. Therefore advice on reducing weight needs to be individualised and balanced with other health considerations.
- **Drink plenty of water** – About six to eight glasses of water (or other low-calorie fluids) a day to prevent dehydration are recommended for the general population, more in warm weather or with increased activity. However, in advanced stages of CKD, fluid (and salt) restriction may be necessary to treat fluid retention in association with diuretics. Most people on dialysis require a fluid restriction (see section on fluid, below).
- **Don't skip breakfast** – It is important to aim to eat regularly and not skip breakfast or other meals. This is good advice for everyone, with or without CKD, regardless of weight. In patients who are underweight or have problems eating enough, attempting more frequent meals or snacks will help to improve overall intake.

The eatwell plate

The eatwell plate (Figure 9.1) is a pictorial representation of the recommended balance of the diet as divided into five main food groups. It is intended to reflect the entire day's intake but can also provide an indication of the balance of a single meal. It can be useful for people with CKD as well as those with other chronic conditions and those who want to reduce their risk of CKD. In more advanced CKD, the relative proportions of each food group may need to be adapted according to symptoms and any therapeutic dietary requirements such as energy supplementation or potassium restriction.

Diet for patients with CKD

The main principles of diet for people with CKD (Figure 9.2) are:

- There is no single diet for CKD – an individual approach is required.
- Optimise nutritional management of any underlying chronic condition such as hypertension, diabetes and obesity.
- Delay progression of CKD by preventing excessive protein intake, control of acidosis and prevention of muscle wasting with adequate energy intake.
- Manage complications of CKD such as hyperkalaemia, fluid retention, hyperphosphataemia and malnutrition.
- Achieve and maintain dietary adequacy and balance, including energy, fibre, macronutrients and micronutrients.

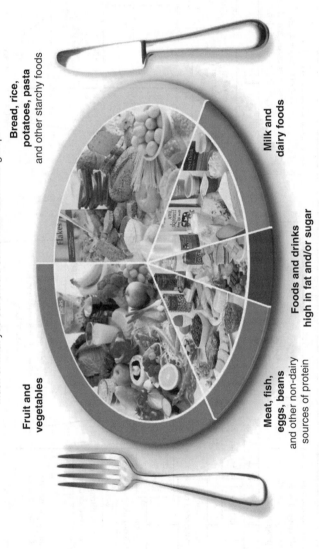

Figure 9.1 The 'eatwell plate'. Crown copyright (Department of Health in association with the Welsh Government, the Scottish Government and the Food Standards Agency in Northern Ireland).

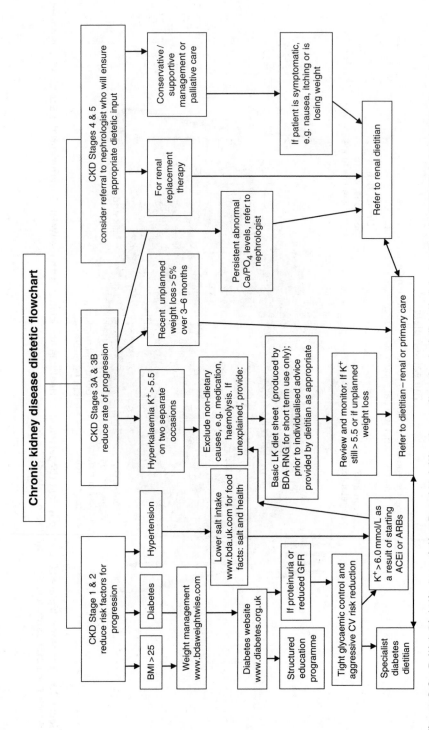

Figure 9.2 British Dietetic Association Renal Nutrition Group flowchart of dietetic intervention in CKD (Renal Nutrition Group).

Diabetes

Diabetes is a major cause of renal impairment in the UK, and dietary treatment of diabetes is essential in both the management and prevention of CKD. Together with appropriate medical management, people with diabetes should be encouraged to follow a healthy diet and lifestyle. The main strategies are summarised in the 2011 Diabetes UK evidence-based nutrition guidelines for the prevention and management of diabetes (Dyson *et al*. 2011).

Glycemic index

Low-glycemic-index (GI) diets have been shown to improve both blood glucose and lipid levels in people with diabetes. The GI is a ranking of carbohydrates according to the extent to which they raise blood glucose levels after eating (Brand-Miller *et al*. 2003). Low-GI foods are more slowly digested and absorbed and cause a more gradual rise in blood glucose and insulin levels. Foods with a high GI are those which are rapidly digested and absorbed. It is also thought that foods with a lower GI are beneficial for weight management, because they help control appetite and delay hunger.

Strategies for managing diabetes include:

- regular carbohydrate-containing meals
- promote lower-GI choices
- maintain a healthy weight
- regular physical activity
- avoid foods high in added sugar
- encourage fruit and vegetables (within any potassium restriction if applicable)
- avoid saturated fat and choose unsaturated fats instead

Hypertension

Hypertension is both a cause and an effect of CKD. A low-salt diet, together with other lifestyle measures, will assist in reducing blood pressure and managing CKD (Sacks *et al*. 2001).

Lifestyle strategies for reducing hypertension include:

- aim for a healthy weight (body mass index 20–25 kg/m²)
- follow a low-salt diet – ideally less than 100 mmol/day
- limit alcohol consumption – less than three units per day for men and less than two units per day for women
- aim for regular exercise – 30 minutes of physical activity such as brisk walking at least three times each week
- include fruit and vegetables daily – aim for five portions per day (or maximum permitted on low-potassium diet if applicable)
- follow a diet low in saturated fat

Low-salt diet

Many patients find it difficult to follow a low-salt diet. Hidden salt contributes to the majority of a patient's salt intake. In the UK people eat around 9 g of salt each day, and much of the excess salt comes from processed foods and ready-made meals. About a quarter comes from the salt we add to meals ourselves. Patients should be advised to avoid added salt and to choose lower salt options whenever possible. Note that potassium-containing salt substitutes such as LoSalt and PanSalt should be avoided by those with CKD.

Practical advice to reduce salt intake:

- It takes time to adjust to the taste of a lower salt diet – allow at least 6–8 weeks.
- Avoid adding salt to meals.
- Use other flavourings such as pepper, lemon, garlic, herbs and spices in place of salty items such as stock cubes, gravy granules and bottled sauces.
- Add only a little, if any, salt to the food when cooking.
- Eat plain or roast meats instead of processed and cured meats such as bacon, sausages and tinned meats.
- Avoid instant noodles and packet and tinned soups.
- Cook with fresh foods as often as possible rather than relying on ready-made or convenience foods.
- Choose low-salt or unsalted options when buying tinned and packaged foods.
- Avoid salty snacks such as crisps, salted crackers, popcorn or salted nuts.
- Read food labels. In sandwiches and packaged meals aim for less than 0.5 g sodium (1.25 g salt) per meal. To convert from sodium to salt multiply the amount by 2.5.

Obesity

Obesity is defined as BMI >30 kg/m². A weight loss of 5–10% can result in improved blood pressure and improved insulin sensitivity. A realistic weight-loss target is approximately 0.5–1.0 kg (1–2 lb) per week. Weight loss greater than this can lead to loss of muscle rather than fat, and unintentional weight loss should be avoided for the same reason. Physical activity should be encouraged, with discussion of safety and barriers to exercise as well as the choice, timing and frequency of exercise.

In general, patients with CKD should be advised to aim for a BMI within the healthy range of 20–25 kg/m², with some variation according to ethnicity. For some groups of CKD patients, such as the more infirm, the elderly and those with more advanced CKD, the need for adequate nutritional intake may override any concerns about overweight. Malnutrition does occur in the obese and is often more difficult to diagnose, delaying treatment. Moreover, a higher BMI is associated with decreased mortality risk in individuals on haemodialysis and a BMI above 23 kg/m² is recommended (Fouque *et al.* 2007). Therefore advice on weight loss needs to be carefully considered in the context of other health priorities.

Nutrients

Protein

The requirement for protein in CKD has often been an area of controversy. Previous advice focused on very strict protein restrictions for the preservation of renal function. The Modification of Diet in Renal Disease trial (Klahr *et al.* 1994), although inconclusive, found that protein intake appeared to have only a minimal effect, if any, on decline in renal function. Furthermore, it is known that patients may spontaneously reduce their protein intake and therefore increase their risk of malnutrition with declining renal function. Current guidelines therefore suggest a moderate protein intake of 0.75–1.0 g of protein per kg (Wright & Jones 2010). This is in fact similar to the advice for the general population. Patients with anorexia, nausea, taste aversions and other barriers to adequate intake will require close monitoring and active encouragement to increase protein intake via food or nutritional supplements. An adequate energy intake is also essential.

Potassium

Declining renal excretion of potassium leads to adaptation by the gut to increase intestinal losses. However, as renal disease progresses, serum potassium levels will rise, depending on dietary intake and other factors. Where possible, the other causes of hyperkalaemia should be corrected to limit the need for dietary intervention.

Non-dietary causes of hyperkalaemia in CKD include:

- medications – including angiotensin converting enzyme inhibitors (ACE inhibitors), angiotensin receptor blockers (ARBs), spironolactone, beta-blockers, non-steroidal anti-inflammatory drugs (NSAIDs) and other contributing drug therapies
- catabolic state as a result of trauma or weight loss (muscle wasting)
- acidosis (check and correct bicarbonate levels)
- heavy exercise
- blood transfusions
- under-dialysis
- constipation (reduced gut losses)

Hyperkalaemia can lead to cardiac arrhythmias and even cardiac arrest. An overzealous approach to potassium restriction can be a problem due to an understandable fear of the worst possible outcome. However, potassium is present in a wide variety of foods including fruit, vegetables, meat and milk, and any intervention needs to be done so as to minimise the effect on choice, palatability and intake of micro- and macronutrients. The aim of the diet is to keep levels stable within safe limits, preventing any sudden increase in serum potassium levels. See Table 9.1 for reference ranges. Patients need to be aware

Table 9.1 Reference ranges for blood potassium levels.

CKD	3.5–5.3 mmol/L (or local normal values)
Haemodialysis	4.0–6.0 mmol/L (level taken immediately before midweek dialysis session)

Renal Association Guidelines (UK).

of those foods that have particularly high potassium content. It is not usually necessary for patients to completely avoid all such foods to achieve adequate control, but they will require advice on levels of intake and suitable substitutions where possible.

There is no need to avoid all fruit and vegetables, as this directly contradicts healthy eating guidelines in removing many beneficial components of the diet. Instead, individuals can be advised to select lower-potassium fruit and vegetables and to adapt cooking methods (Jackson *et al.* 2006). Control of high-potassium drinks and snacks is important, as they may otherwise be taken in inconsistent amounts and cause unstable serum levels.

A low-potassium diet should be regularly reviewed to assess the appropriate level of restriction, particularly in response to medication changes or in situations such as inter-current illness. In the case of anorexia or poor intake for other reasons, a referral to the dietitian for a review of the potassium restriction will help to prioritise energy and other nutrients.

Treatment of hyperkalaemia

Suggested first-line potassium restriction for outpatients with hyperkalaemia includes:

- Avoid all salt substitutes which are potassium-based, such as Selora, LoSalt and PanSalt.
- Choose lower-potassium drinks such as water, fizzy drinks, flavoured water, squash (not high juice varieties), tea and herbal tea. Limit milk to half a pint (280 mL) daily. Limit coffee to 1-2 cups day. Avoid or limit these potassium-rich drinks: fruit and vegetable juices, chocolate and malted drinks.
- Choose lower-potassium snacks such as plain, jam, cream-filled biscuits and cakes, doughnuts, crumpets, crackers, croissants, boiled sweets and regular or sugar-free mints. Eat fewer high-potassium snacks such as crisps, nuts, Bombay mix, chocolate, toffee, fudge and liquorice.
- Have a moderate fruit and vegetable and salad intake of a total of 4-5 portions daily. A portion is about 80 g or about one handful of fruit or 2-3 tablespoons of cooked vegetables or salad. Some are particularly high in potassium, so avoid or eat less of the following: bananas, avocado, okra, spinach, all dried fruit and tomato puree.
- Adapt cooking methods to remove some of the potassium. Boil potatoes, yams and other vegetables in plenty of water and throw away the water before eating or cooking further. This includes before frying or roasting or

before adding to stews, soups and curries. Avoid microwaving or steaming vegetables. There is no need to soak vegetables before boiling.

Low-potassium advice for hospitalised patients

Hospitalised patients are even more vulnerable to the side effects of a restricted diet as there are multiple barriers to adequate food intake. It is particularly important to consider non-dietary causes of hyperkalaemia and to avoid compromising energy and protein status. Excess potassium often derives from sources other than the hospital menu, such as chocolates, nuts, dried fruit, fresh fruit, juices, coffee and milky drinks. Patients can be advised on suitable alternatives such as lower-potassium fruit, plain, jam and cream biscuits and cakes, tea and fruit squashes. The hospital menu should provide lower-potassium vegetable and fruit choices and alternatives to potato such as rice, bread, pasta and noodles where possible. Potassium-based salt substitutes must not be given. For patients requiring nutrition support, a referral to the ward dietitian is recommended for specialist advice. Powdered milkshakes, soups and other products with high milk content are generally to be avoided.

Renal replacement and potassium

Haemodialysis (HD) is an effective method of potassium removal. However, there is a risk of excessive accumulation of potassium between dialysis sessions. Therefore, in many patients (but not all) some dietary control of potassium is necessary to limit the peak potassium level between haemodialysis sessions within safe limits, as defined by the Renal Association (Table 9.1). Lower pre-dialysis potassium levels, even those within the normal range, may indicate an over-restrictive diet regimen or inadequate dietary intake as a whole and an increased risk of malnutrition. Individualising and reviewing dietary advice remains essential in maintaining a balanced and adequate nutritional intake.

Peritoneal dialysis (PD) removes potassium effectively on a daily basis, so the need for potassium restriction is less common and often there is a risk of hypokalaemia in patients with an inadequate intake. On starting PD, patients can often relax dietary potassium restrictions and may even need specific advice on a high-potassium diet. This should be given in the context of the whole diet, including protein and energy and other nutrients, and optimising fruit and vegetables, rather than just considering potassium as an isolated nutrient.

Renal transplant patients may develop hyperkalaemia with delayed or inadequate graft function or as a result of immunosuppressive drug regimens and will need to follow a potassium restriction until these issues are resolved.

Phosphate

Phosphate retention is a consequence of a reduction in glomerular filtration rate (GFR) and can occur before any rise in serum phosphate levels is apparent. It has a detrimental effect on calcium homeostasis and parathyroid hormone

Table 9.2 Reference ranges for blood phosphate levels.

CKD stage 3B–5	0.9–1.5 mmol/L
Dialysis	1.1–1.7 mmol/L

Renal Association Guidelines (UK).

(PTH) production, leading to the development of CKD mineral and bone disorder (CKD-MBD). This is characterised by a low serum calcium, high serum phosphate and high PTH levels in CKD stage 4 and 5. A reduction in the production of the active form of vitamin D (1,25-dihydroxycholecalciferol or calcitriol) in the kidneys contributes to hypocalcaemia and hyperparathyroidism.

Dietary phosphate restriction is important in phosphate control, but the stage at which this should start is unclear. It is usually initiated once phosphate levels start to rise above normal. However, limits on phosphate intake at an earlier stage may be beneficial (Ash *et al.* 2006). Table 9.2 refers to reference ranges.

Low-phosphate diet

A low-phosphate diet is central to the management of CKD-MBD (KDIGO 2009). High-phosphate foods include meat, fish, eggs, nuts and protein-rich dairy foods such as milk, cheese and yoghurt. The challenge is to ensure that the low-phosphate diet remains balanced in terms of protein, energy and other nutrients and is compatible with chronic disease prevention and any other dietary regimens. To avoid compromising protein intake it is usual to limit foods with a higher phosphate content relative to their protein content such as dairy foods, offal, shellfish and oily fish (Fouque *et al.* 2007).

To address concerns about phosphate retention, patients in earlier stages of CKD and who have normal phosphate levels can be advised to follow national healthy eating guidelines. This provides a guide to moderate protein portions and can help to curb excess phosphate intakes while addressing chronic disease management and risk. High intakes of dairy foods should be avoided.

Phosphate-binding medication

Phosphate binders are used in combination with a low-phosphate diet to reduce the absorption of phosphate into the body (KDIGO 2009). They bind with dietary phosphate in the gut so that it is excreted in the stool. Calcium-based binders are the most commonly used, as they are cheap and effective, but there are some concerns about the effects of excess calcium absorption with larger doses. Alternatives include binders based on sevelamer (a polymer resin), lanthanum (a rare metal) and aluminium, although the last is now seldom used because of the risk of aluminium toxicity.

Patients and their carers need to be aware of the need to match administration of binders with the quantity and timing of phosphate intake. Binders should be taken with or before phosphate-containing meals or snacks. This will optimise their action and reduce the risk of side effects such as hypercalcaemia.

Low-phosphate diet: main principles

The main principles of a low-phosphate diet include:

- Dairy and eggs – relatively high phosphate-to-protein ratios – allowances set for milk, cheese, milk products and eggs. Avoid tinned and dried milk powder.
- Meat and fish – limit processed meat products, offal, shellfish, oily fish and fish with edible bones (such as whitebait, anchovies, tinned fish and dried or ground whole fish). Other meat and fish as usual but take a binder if prescribed.
- Drinks and snacks – limit milky drinks. Limit nuts including coconut. Limit chocolate and gram-flour-based snacks.
- Starchy staples (such as bread, pasta, rice, potatoes), fruit, vegetables, herbs and spices are mostly unrestricted.
- Sugar, jam, honey, fats, oils and cream are low in phosphate and can be taken as usual.
- Correct choice, dose and timing of phosphate binder in relation to intake.

Hypophosphataemia

In dialysis patients, low phosphate levels can be an indicator of low phosphate (and inevitably protein) intake as phosphate continues to be dialysed regardless. An excess dose of phosphate binders in relation to phosphate intake can also cause hypophosphataemia. A serum phosphate level below the recommended range should prompt a review of binders and adequacy of nutritional intake as a whole, particularly protein.

Fluid

Fluid management is important for cardiovascular health. Although multifactorial, fluid overload is known to be a significant precursor in the development of left ventricular hypertension and increased mortality in people with kidney disease. Patients at all stages of CKD find fluid management confusing and will benefit from clear explanations of the concepts involved. Most patients on dialysis are fluid restricted, and they often find this one of the most challenging aspects of the diet.

Establishing a fluid allowance

Patients need to be advised on an individualised fluid allowance, and this should be reviewed regularly. Patients on dialysis will usually experience a reduction in urine output over time. They should be aware of their 24-hour urine output volume and how to measure this on a regular basis, or as clinically indicated.

Helpful strategies for patients on fluid restrictions include:

- Know your fluid allowance.
- Know your dry (or target) weight.

- Know the guidelines for inter-dialytic weight gain (haemodialysis).
- Spread fluid over the day.
- Limit salt and salty foods to reduce thirst.
- Limit other foods that are found to increase thirst such as very spicy, astringent or powdery/dry foods.
- Try sucking an ice cube instead of a cold drink.
- Snacking on fruit (within any fruit allowance) can help to reduce thirst.
- Choose small cups or glasses.
- Try sucking on sugar-free boiled sweets, mints or chewing on gum between meals.
- Practise good dental hygiene - including regular brushing and use of suitable mouthwash.
- Sip drinks to make them last longer.
- Add lemon or lime wedges to drinks.
- Limit high-fluid foods such as soup, gravy, sauces and jelly.
- When having casseroles, curry, stews, main-course soups and other similar dishes, drain off the liquid before serving.

Table 9.3 shows the approximate volumes of a range of containers for fluids.

Table 9.3 Volume guide (approximate amounts).

Mug	250 mL
Teacup	180 mL
Espresso cup	80 mL
Medium wine glass	250 mL
Water glass	200–300 mL
Ice cube	15–20 mL
1 tablespoon	15 mL

Vitamins and minerals

Vitamin supplementation in renal patients is controversial, owing to a lack of evidence to support its long-term use. In the UK practice differs from one renal unit to another.

- **Water-soluble vitamins should be supplemented** - Water-soluble vitamin supplementation may be necessary because of factors such as dialysis losses (Wright & Jones 2010), dietary restrictions, observed low plasma vitamins and poor oral intake in the population. Additionally, water-soluble vitamins are linked with homocysteine levels and anaemia management.
- **Vitamin D supplements are generally recommended** - Vitamin D deficiency is widespread in the general population. In patients with CKD,

vitamin D_3 should be corrected as necessary in the standard manner. With CKD there is impaired renal synthesis to the 'active' form, 1,25-dihydroxy-cholecalciferol, and a vitamin D analogue such as calcitriol, alfacalcidol or paracalcitrol is usually required. Dosing is according to serum levels of calcium, phosphate, PTH and other bone markers, which must be regularly monitored.

- **Vitamin A supplements should be avoided** – An excessive intake of vitamin A is associated with elevated serum calcium levels. General multivitamins and supplements containing high quantities of vitamin A, such as cod liver oil, should be avoided.

Acidosis and nutrition

In CKD, acidosis occurs because the kidneys are less able to synthesise ammonia and excrete hydrogen ions. Correction of acidosis may lead to improvement in nutritional status and bone health. Treatment with sodium bicarbonate may also help to delay the progression of CKD and does not appear to have an adverse effect on blood pressure (de Brito-Ashurst et al. 2009). National recommendations suggest maintaining bicarbonate levels above 22 mmol/L (Wright & Jones 2010).

Haemodialysis

Standard haemodialysis (HD) takes place three times each week. Due to its intermittent nature there is a need to limit accumulation of waste products between sessions, especially fluid and potassium. The British Dietetic Association (BDA) Renal Nutrition Group recommends the European Best Practice Guidelines on Nutrition to provide guidance for nutrients other than protein requirements (BDA Renal Nutrition Group 2011) (Table 9.4).

Protein and energy

Patients undergoing HD are at high risk of malnutrition. Causes include multiple comorbidities and older age, socioeconomic issues, depression, chronic inflammation and poor intake due to time spent travelling and waiting for treatment, or due to multiple dietary restrictions. An adequate energy intake in combination with sufficient protein is essential to achieve an optimal metabolic balance (BDA Renal Nutrition Group 2011).

Patients with a normal or higher BMI may still have inadequate protein and micronutrient intakes, especially if they are inactive, because of the difficulty in selecting a sufficiently high-quality, nutrient-rich diet. It is important to encourage patients to be as active as possible in their daily life.

Table 9.4 Summary of the European and British guidelines and recommendations.

Nutrient	Guideline and recommendation
Protein	1.1 g/kg oedema-free body weight/day where energy intake is adequate (BDA recommendation)
Energy	30–40 kcal/kg IBW/day in a clinically stable chronic haemodialysis patient, adjusted for age, gender and the best estimate of physical activity level
Potassium	50–70 mmol (1950–2730 mg) or 1 mmol/kg IBW/ day in patients with a pre-dialysis serum potassium >6 mmol/L
Phosphate	800–1000 mg phosphate/day
Sodium	No more than 80–100 mmol (2000–2300 mg) sodium or 5–6 g (75 mg/kg BW) of sodium chloride per day
Fluid	Daily fluid intake of 500–1000 mL in addition to volume equal to daily urine output. Individual fluid allowances need to be adapted for patients living in warmer climates, during periods of hot weather, working in hot environments and as a result of clinical conditions such as high fever. Inter-dialytic weight gain (IDWG) should not exceed 4–4.5% of dry body weight.

IBW, ideal body weight.
Data from Fouque *et al*, 2007; BDA Renal Nutrition Group, 2011.

Fluid and salt

A restricted fluid intake is required to limit accumulation of fluid between HD sessions to a maximum of 4–4.5% dry body weight (usually 2–3 kg). Control of fluid will improve blood pressure control and tolerance of HD, reduce tissue oedema and reduce the risk of left ventricular hypertrophy and breathlessness. All fluid-restricted patients require a salt restriction to minimise thirst and fluid retention.

Potassium and phosphate

Many HD patients need to limit potassium intake to control potassium accumulation between dialysis sessions. Fruit and vegetable intakes should be optimised within the restriction to maintain micronutrient and fibre intake. Phosphate is removed by HD, but patients will usually need to limit phosphate intake and take phosphate binders for adequate phosphate control. It is important to maintain adequate protein intake. Patients with low serum phosphate should have their binder dosage reduced and diet reviewed for overall nutritional adequacy.

Peritoneal dialysis

The BDA Renal Nutrition Group recommends the 2000 KDOQI National Kidney Foundation clinical practice guidelines for nutrition in chronic renal failure to guide practice in areas other than protein and energy requirements (BDA Renal Nutrition Group 2011).

Protein and energy

Most PD fluids are glucose-based, and approximately 30–70% of the glucose will be absorbed, depending on factors such as the dialysis prescription and individual peritoneal membrane characteristics. This will provide an energy load of about 250–500 kcal for most patients. The glucose absorption will also directly affect diabetes control. Exposure of the peritoneal membrane to higher-strength glucose solutions should be minimised because of the increased risk of premature technique failure.

During PD there are incidental losses of protein of approximately 5–15 g/day depending on individual membrane characteristics and dialysis regimen. The British Dietetic Association recommends a minimum protein intake of 1.0–1.2 g/kg oedema-free body weight per day. There is an emphasis on the need for an adequate total energy intake (from diet and dialysate) of 30–35 kcal/kg oedema-free body weight per day (BDA Renal Nutrition Group 2011). Despite the additional calorie source, malnutrition is widespread due to the general factors related to CKD and its treatment and additional PD-specific causes. These include peritonitis and other infections and abdominal discomfort due to the presence of dialysis fluid. For some patients the peritoneal absorption of glucose can be a useful extra source of energy. For others it represents 'empty calories' and causes excess weight gain and a relative deficit of protein and micronutrients. Regular dietary assessment and advice on achieving a high-quality, nutrient-rich diet are essential. It is important to encourage patients to be as active as possible in their daily life and to advise on suitable forms of exercise.

Fluid and salt

Control of fluid intake will help to reduce reliance on high-strength glucose solutions which remove more water but increase glucose absorption. Recommended fluid allowance is approximately 800 mL in addition to a volume equal to the 24-hour urine output (Ash et al. 2006). This will vary according to individual peritoneal membrane characteristics and dialysis regimen, as well as climate and clinical condition. Patients following a fluid restriction will require advice on salt restriction to reduce thirst and fluid retention.

Potassium and phosphate

Most PD regimens remove potassium efficiently on a daily basis. Patients with low potassium intakes are at risk from hypokalaemia due to the continuous removal of potassium. Patients may require education on increasing potassium in their diet. Many PD patients will need to limit phosphate intake, and will require phosphate binders for adequate phosphate control. However, hypophosphataemia is a risk in patients with poor intakes, especially if dietary protein is lacking.

Fibre

Prevention of constipation is important for functioning PD. Patients should be encouraged to have adequate fibre in their diet with plenty of fruit and vegetables within any potassium restriction if this applies. Soluble fibre supplements may be beneficial in preventing constipation without the side effects of stimulant laxatives (Sutton *et al.* 2007).

Transplant

A successful kidney transplant gives a patient increased dietary freedom. Diet plays an important role in preventing and managing obesity, diabetes, cardiovascular disease, hypertension, dyslipidaemia and bone disease, which can all occur in the transplant recipient. Despite a renal transplant, most patients will still have a degree of CKD, which can make them particularly complex to manage. There is little research regarding diet and outcomes in this population, and many dietary recommendations are therefore similar to those for healthy individuals.

Dyslipidamia is present in approximately 60% of renal transplant recipients and is strongly associated with cardiovascular disease (GMCT 2008). Immunosuppressive regimes, together with pre-existing dyslipidaemia and lifestyle factors, can contribute to abnormal lipid profiles.

Hypertension is a risk factor for cardiovascular disease and can adversely affect graft survival. Patients should be encouraged to continue with a low-salt diet after a transplant. Additionally, alcohol consumption should be based on recommendations for the general population, because of its influence on cardiovascular disease.

Patients should be made aware of the risk of weight gain after a renal transplant. This is multifactorial and associated with increased dietary flexibility and improved wellbeing. Steroid use is also known to stimulate appetite. The majority of the weight gained tends to occur in the first year and can be as high at 35% (GMCT 2008). Obesity is associated with poor graft survival and contributes to hypertension, diabetes and dyslipidaemia. New-onset diabetes after transplantation (NODAT) is associated with graft failure and cardiovascular disease and has been reported to affect 20% of patients at one year post transplant. Immunosuppressive regimens, in addition to traditional risk factors such as age, ethnicity and family history, will influence NODAT risk.

During the initial few weeks following a kidney transplant, patients should be encouraged to take a higher-protein diet, particularly if graft function is delayed and the patient continues to need dialysis. Additionally, a higher protein intake promotes wound healing. A protein intake of 1.3 g/kg in the first four weeks is suggested. Subsequently, stable patients should be encouraged to have a moderate protein intake in line with general healthy eating guidelines (GMCT 2008).

The management of bone disease is complex in kidney disease, and prior to transplantation there are likely to be several bone health abnormalities.

The risk of fracture is higher in this group than in the general population. Factors contributing to poorer bone metabolism include poor calcium absorption related to steroid use, hypophosphatemia, particularly in the first few months post transplant, and abnormal vitamin D metabolism (GMCT 2008). Patients should be encouraged take a high-phosphate diet, as early as possible after a renal transplant to help correct hypophosphataemia. Some patients will require oral phosphate supplementation if levels cannot be normalised with a high-phosphate diet and if they are symptomatic. However, if supplemented late in the post-transplant phase, hyperparathyroidism can be worsened (GMCT 2008). See the section on phosphate, above, for practical suggestions.

Calcium intake should follow guidelines for the general population. Physical activity, particularly weight-bearing activity, is important for bone health and should be encouraged. Vitamin D supplements (or analogue) have been shown to have a favourable effect on bone mineral density.

Establishing a fluid goal as early as possible is important. Many patients have been so used to restricting fluid intake that they can find drinking sufficient fluid difficult.

There is thought to be an increased risk of food-borne illnesses such as listeriosis due to immunosuppressant medications, particularly in the early stages after a transplant when doses are higher. Patients are advised on their vulnerability regarding food-borne illnesses and on standard food safety and hygiene, including storage and preparation of raw and cooked food.

When should a kidney transplant patient see a dietitian?

The recently published Evidenced Based Practice Guidelines for the Nutritional Management of Adult Kidney Transplant Recipients (GMCT 2008) suggest that patients should be seen routinely by a dietitian as soon as practicable after a transplant and followed up monthly for the first three months. An annual review is recommended thereafter. Interim referral and review may be required for various reasons including management of comorbidities and symptoms as they occur.

Summary for diet in renal transplant recipients

- Eat a diet based on the eatwell plate which is high in vegetables, fruit and whole grains (Figure 9.1).
- Have a diet low in saturated fat. Use fats which are based on unsaturated fats such as olive oil, margarines and sunflower oil.
- Continue to follow a low-salt diet.
- Aim for a moderate protein intake. However, aim to include oily fish regularly.
- Choose low-fat dairy foods.
- Use a vitamin D supplement as appropriate for the individual.
- Drink alcohol in moderation.
- Aim for regular physical activity.
- Ensure adequate fluid intake.
- Follow good food hygiene practices.

Malnutrition, nutritional assessment and intervention

Malnutrition is widespread in patients with CKD, especially in its more advanced stages, and can have a significant impact on morbidity and mortality (Fouque *et al.* 2007). Malnutrition is also referred to more specifically as protein-energy wasting (PEW). It can develop quickly and, once established, is difficult to treat.

Causes of malnutrition in CKD

There are many possible causes of PEW in CKD. Factors include increased requirements, increased losses and multiple barriers to intake. These vary from a non-specific loss of appetite, chronic infections and dialysis protein losses to the economic, social and psychological implications of a chronic illness (Table 9.5).

Table 9.5 Causes of malnutrition in CKD.

Cause of malnutrition	Inadequate intake	Increased requirements
Examples of contributing factors	Socioeconomic, including social isolation, financial difficulties, inability to work	Inflammation
	Psychological, such as depression, anxiety and stress	Infection, including dialysis-specific infections such as HD line sepsis and PD peritonitis
	Uraemic symptoms such as anorexia, acid reflux, nausea, vomiting, taste changes, food aversions especially with under-dialysis or delayed dialysis	Increased protein catabolism associated with factors such as energy deficit, low activity levels, increased infections, acidosis, insulin resistance and hyperparathyroidism
	Pharmaceutical, including polypharmacy and drug-related side effects	
	Inappropriate, unbalanced or inadequately monitored 'therapeutic' diets	
	Treatment-related, including time and effort attending the HD unit or doing PD and early satiety with PD fluid in situ	Drug side effects
	Recurrent/prolonged hospital admissions	Increased losses, including proteinuria and protein losses on HD and PD
	Anaemia, inter-current illnesses, physical infirmity or disability	
	Comorbidities such as cancer, HIV, gastrointestinal disease	Comorbidities

Nutritional assessment

The diagnosis of malnutrition in renal patients can be particularly challenging, as many indices of nutritional status may be directly altered by renal failure or other disease processes. There is currently no single method of nutritional assessment that is considered ideal, but using a combination of approaches is recommended (Wright & Jones 2010).

Anthropometric assessment

Anthropometry includes the measurement of height, weight, circumference of various body parts and skin fold thickness at different sites. The procedures are generally simple, inexpensive, safe and non-invasive. However, certain aspects of kidney disease, such as fluid retention, can affect their use and interpretation.

Fluid retention may mask loss of muscle or fat mass. The best estimation of oedema-free weight should be used for nutritional assessment and calculations such as BMI (weight/height2). In dialysis patients the current 'dry' or 'target' weight should be obtained from the renal unit records.

There is a lack of knowledge generally amongst patients regarding malnutrition, and improving awareness of weight changes can help. However, this is not always easy. Those with fluid retention may report that they feel fat or overweight – sometimes to the extent that they will intentionally limit food intake and exacerbate PEW. Conversely, a resolution of oedema may be reported as 'weight loss'. It is useful to obtain a weight history to quantify and explain changes in body weight over time. It is important to clarify weight terminology such as dry weight, target weight and ideal weight. Patients can be advised to self-monitor and report other indicators such as upper-body wasting, anorexia and reduced intake.

Waist and hip circumference measurements can be used to assess for central obesity and cardiovascular disease risk unless the abdomen is distended, for example by the presence of peritoneal fluid, ascites or polycystic organs.

Measurements of triceps skin fold and mid-upper arm circumference can be used to assess and monitor local changes in muscle and fat in individual patients over time. These measurements can be affected by fluid status and should ideally be taken post-haemodialysis or when the subject is at a dry weight. Handgrip dynamometry measures grip strength, and in renal patients it has been found to correlate well with lean body mass and have prognostic value (Wang et al. 2005).

The right side is preferred for upper-arm anthropometry and handgrip measurements, as this is consistent with standard reference data. In practice, it will need to be the side without vascular access, dressings or other obstacles. Comparison of measurements with reference tables can be difficult and needs to take into account any differences in methodology, age and other selection criteria of the reference population. In practice an individual's measurements will be taken and compared over time to monitor progress.

Biochemical assessment

Serum albumin concentration is a less reliable indicator of nutritional status. Low albumin levels may be related to fluid overload, inflammation, sepsis or other factors and require medical investigation. Conversely, normal albumin levels do not preclude a diagnosis of malnutrition. C-reactive protein (CRP) increases with the acute-phase response and can help in interpreting albumin levels (Wright & Jones 2010).

Subjective global assessment

Subjective Global Assessment (SGA) is widely recommended in renal patients (Wright & Jones 2010). Requiring minimal resources and modest training for the doctor, nurse or dietitian, the SGA combines a short clinical history with a physical examination. This results in an overall impression of nutritional status without the need for precise body composition analysis. This subjective classification of the patient by nutritional status has been shown to correlate well with future morbidity and mortality (Table 9.6). The Patient-Generated Subjective Global Assessment (PG-SGA) has been developed to include a numerical score as well as an overall subjective rating. It is also validated for use with renal patients.

Nutritional screening

Nutritional screening is undertaken to detect those individuals within a group who are at risk of malnutrition and to determine if a more detailed assessment or other intervention is needed. Because of the increased risk of malnutrition

Table 9.6 Subjective Global Assessment (SGA) tool outline.

History

Weight/weight change – using best estimation of dry weight

Dietary intake – change/no change

Gastrointestinal symptoms (anorexia, nausea, vomiting, diarrhoea) – frequency/duration

Functional capacity

Disease state/comorbidities as related to nutritional needs

Physical examination
- Loss of subcutaneous fat
- Muscle wasting
- Oedema
- Ascites

Overall SGA rating: A, very mild to well-nourished; B, mild to moderately malnourished; C, severely malnourished.
Jeejeebhoy, K. (2012). Subjective Global Assessment: A highly reliable nutritional assessment tool. Available at: http://subjectiveglobalassessment.com/.

with CKD it should be integral to the role of all health professionals caring for these patients (Wright & Jones 2010). Generic methods, such as the Malnutrition Universal Screening Tool (MUST), are in widespread use. However, these may not be fully applicable to patients with CKD, and work to develop renal-specific malnutrition screening tools is ongoing (Wright & Jones 2010).

Renal Association recommended frequency of screening for under-nutrition in CKD (Wright & Jones 2010):

- Weekly for inpatients.
- 2-3-monthly for outpatients with eGFR <20 but not on dialysis.
- Within one month of commencement of dialysis then 6-8 weeks later.
- 4-6-monthly for stable haemodialysis patients.
- 4-6-monthly for stable peritoneal dialysis patients.
- Screening may need to occur more frequently if risk of under-nutrition is increased, for example by inter-current illness.

Dietary treatment of malnutrition

(1) Thorough **Assessment** of diet and weight, including weight history.
(2) **Identification** of barriers to meeting nutritional requirements.
(3) Consider **referral** to other members of the specialist team, for instance a renal social worker, nephrologist or psychologist, for specific issues such as financial or emotional difficulties, medication review or medical assessment.
(4) **Treatment** with dietary modification and individualised advice.
(5) **Ongoing review.**

First-line strategies for improving intake (dietetic referral is recommended if the patient has diabetes or is on a low-potassium, low-phosphate or other restricted diet):

- Increase frequency of intake: encourage small regular meals and snacks at 1-2-hourly intervals.
- Increase snacks : examples include, toast, crackers, biscuits, cakes.
- Increase energy and/or protein density by adding value to existing foods. Examples include:
  - adding additional fat and oil in cooking
  - extra butter or margarine on toast or bread
  - adding cream to sauces, on fruit and desserts
  - adding extra diced meat, egg, tofu, tinned fish or grated cheese to existing dishes such as rice or mashed potatoes
- Reduce bulky/nutrient poor foods such as soup, salads and fizzy drinks.

At more advanced stages of malnutrition, or if dietary manipulation is insufficient or not possible, manufactured oral nutritional supplements can be considered in consultation with a dietitian. Standard 1.5 kcal/mL complete supplement drinks are commonly used as they are nutritionally balanced and come in a wide variety of flavours to increase acceptance. However, more specialist products (higher protein and energy, low volume and electrolytes) are often required. Over-the-counter supplements may not be suitable for CKD patients because of volume and electrolyte content.

At times enteral or parenteral feeds may be indicated for renal patients who are unable to meet their nutritional requirements with oral diet and nutritional supplements. A referral to a dietitian will be required.

Inter-dialytic parenteral nutrition (IDPN)

Inter-dialytic parenteral (IDPN) nutrition is given via the venous return during haemodialysis. It typically supplies up to 1000 kcal, 7 g nitrogen per session but is usually incomplete in terms of vitamins and minerals. It cannot be used as the sole method of nutrition support, is relatively expensive and is not without risks such as hyperglycaemia. The decision to use IDPN should be a multidisciplinary one only once all options for enteral nutrition, including tube feeding, have been exhausted.

Conclusion

Meeting the nutritional needs of people with CKD is clinically challenging, and patients typically have complex nutritional needs. CKD includes a spectrum of health states, and it is important to ensure that the diet is nutritionally balanced, acceptable and safe, wherever the patient is on his or her illness pathway. Renal nutrition can often seem confusing, and clinicians should provide consistent, individualised and evidence-based information and advice. Dietary treatment is essential to manage comorbidities and electrolyte and fluid balance, and to reduce the risk of malnutrition. A multi-professional approach and regular nutrition screening and assessment are recommended.

References

Ash, S., Campbell, K., Maclaughlin, H. et al. (2006) Evidence based practice guidelines for the nutritional management of chronic kidney disease. Nutrition and Dietetics, 63, S33-45.

BDA Renal Nutrition Group (2011) Evidence Based Dietetic Guidelines: Protein Requirements of Adults on Haemodialysis and Peritoneal Dialysis. British Dietetic Association, Birmingham.

Brand-Miller, J., Hayne, S., Petocz, P. & Colagiuri, S. (2003) Low-glycemic index diets in the management of diabetes: a meta-analysis of randomized controlled trials. Diabetes Care, 26, 2261-7.

de Brito-Ashurst, I., Varagunam, M., Raftery, M.J. & Yaqoob, M.M. (2009) Bicarbonate supplementation slows progression of ckd and improves nutritional status. Journal of the American Society of Nephrology, 20, 2075-84.

Dyson, P.A., Kelly, T., Deakin, T. *et al.* (2011) Diabetes UK evidence-based nutrition guidelines for the prevention and management of diabetes. *Diabetic Medicine,* **28**, 1282–8.

Fouque, D., Vennegoor, M., Wee, P.T. *et al.* (2007) ERA-EDTNA European best practice guideline on nutrition. *Nephrology, Dialysis, Transplantation,* **22** (Suppl. 2), 45–87.

GMCT (Renal Services Network) (2008) *Evidence Based Practice Guidelines for the Nutritional Management of Adult Kidney Transplant Recipients.* Greater Metropolitan Clinical Taskforce, Sydney.

Jackson, H., Cassidy, A. & James, G. (2006) *Eating Well with Kidney Failure: a Practical Guide and Cookbook.* Class Publishing, London.

KDIGO (2009) KDIGO clinical practice guideline for the diagnosis, evaluation, prevention, and treatment of chronic kidney disease-mineral and bone disorder (CKD-MBD). *Kidney International,* **76**, s1–132.

KDOQI (National Kidney Foundation Kidney Disease Outcomes Quality Initiative) (2007) KDOQI clinical practice guidelines and clinical practice recommendations for diabetes and chronic kidney disease. *American Journal of Kidney Diseases,* **49** (2 Suppl. 2), S12–154.

Klahr, S., Levey, A.S., Beck, G.J. *et al.* (1994) The effects of dietary protein restriction and blood-pressure control on the progression of chronic renal disease. *New England Journal of Medicine,* **330**, 877–84.

Sacks, F., Svetkey, L., Vollmer, W. *et al.* (2001) Effects on blood pressure of reduced dietary sodium and the Dietary Approaches to Stop Hypertension (DASH) Diet. *New England Journal of Medicine,* **334**, 3–10.

Sutton, D., Dumbleton, S. & Allaway, C. (2007) Can increased dietary fibre reduce laxative requirement in peritoneal dialysis patients? *Journal of Renal Care,* **33**, 174–8.

Wang, A., Sea, M., Ho, Z. *et al.* (2005) Evaluation of handgrip strength as a nutritional marker and prognostic indicator in peritoneal dialysis patients. *American Journal of Clinical Nutrition,* **81**, 79–86.

Wright, M. & Jones, C. (2010) Clinical practice guidelines on nutrition in CKD, 5th edition. Renal Association. http://www.renal.org/Clinical/GuidelinesSection/NutritionInCKD.aspx (accessed September 2012).

Resources

British Dietetic Association. Food fact sheets. (For printable information sheets on diet and nutrition.) http://www.bda.uk.com/foodfacts (accessed September 2012).

Guy's and St Thomas' NHS Foundation Trust (2011) *Everyday Eating: Tasty Recipes and Helpful Hints for Kidney Patients by Kidney Patients.* http://www.guysandstthomas.nhs.uk/resources/patient-information/kidney/EverydayEating-recipeBookforkidneypatients.pdf (accessed September 2012).

Jackson, H., Cassidy, A. & James, G. (2006) *Eating Well with Kidney Failure: a Practical Guide and Cookbook.* Class Publishing, London (for CKD 4–5).

Jackson, H., Green, C. & James, G. (2009) *Eating Well for Kidney Health: Expert Guidance and Delicious Recipes.* Class Publishing, London (for CKD 1–3).

NHS Choices. Live well. (For general information on healthy eating and lifestyle.) http://www.nhs.uk/livewell (accessed September 2012).

Twomey, V. & McElveen, H. (2010) *Truly Tasty: Over 100 Special Recipes Created by Irelands Top Chefs for Adults Living with Kidney Disease.* Cork University Press, Cork.

Chapter 10

Supportive and Palliative Care for Patients with Advanced Kidney Disease

Sheila Johnston[1], Helen Noble[2] and Rachel Lewis[3]

[1] Royal Free London NHS Foundation Trust, London, UK
[2] Queen's University Belfast, UK
[3] Manchester Business School, The University of Manchester, UK

Introduction

It is estimated that 9% of the English adult population have chronic kidney disease (CKD) stages 3–5. Within this group there is a disproportionate number of older patients, many of whom have other chronic conditions, and there is a 4% risk of reaching stage 5 CKD. Most patients with CKD die from other conditions, usually vascular, but a proportion will die from progressive kidney disease, and a significant number of dialysis-dependent patients will die following a decision to withdraw from dialysis. A growing cohort of palliative patients are those who have advanced CKD, both progressive and stable, who are clinically unsuitable for dialysis, or who have chosen not to have it. The key to providing effective supportive and palliative care to people with CKD is in pre-emptively identifying those likely to need it and ensuring that appropriate systems are in place to meet individual needs as required. Part of this challenge is the heterogeneity of health states in patients with CKD and the uncertainty in patterns of chronic illness progression. The purpose of this chapter is to assist in the identification and management of patients with chronic kidney disease approaching the terminal phase of their lives. It includes references to evidence-based guidelines and pathways of care aimed at the practical organisation and coordination of care as well as symptom management.

Background

Around 45 000 people receive renal replacement therapy (RRT) in the UK, of whom just under half have a kidney transplant and the rest are on dialysis. Most are older adults and have at least one other chronic condition. Consequently mortality in this population is high, and patients receiving dialysis have a much shorter life expectancy than a comparable age group in the general population. As Table 10.1 shows, the chance of surviving 1–10 years on dialysis is age-dependent.

Chronic kidney disease is a life-limiting illness, but nonetheless most patients die from other causes. Table 10.2 illustrates the commonest causes of death in patients with kidney disease.

Approximately 15% of older patients opt for a non-dialytic care pathway. These people tend to be those with multiple chronic conditions who may already be frail and require a high degree of health and social support. The evidence to date suggests that for patients starting dialysis in similar health states, dialysis confers no additional benefit in terms of longevity and can often incur a significant burden affecting the patient's quality of

Table 10.1 Percentage chance of surviving 1, 2, 5 and 10 years following commencement of dialysis, depending on the age the patient at start of dialysis (Modified from Stein & Wild 2002).

Age starting dialysis	1 year	2 years	5 years	10 years
<20 years	98%	95%	88%	79%
20–44 years	94%	88%	71%	52%
45–64 years	88%	77%	44%	15%
65–74 years	75%	58%	21%	2%
>74 years	63%	44%	10%	1%

Table 10.2 Common causes of death in patients with CKD (Modified from Stein & Wild 2002).

	Dialysis patients	Transplant patients
Heart disease	42%	30%
Infections	15%	12%
Strokes	12%	12%
Treatment withdrawn	18%	3%
Cancer	6%	34%
Other	6%	9%

life. The aim of management is to ensure that patients receive the appropriate care and support irrespective of where that is delivered. This requires a regular assessment of need, ongoing discussions with patients and their families, supported decision making and coordination across care providers.

Identifying patients with CKD approaching the end of life

As with other chronic conditions, identifying when a patient with advanced kidney disease is approaching the end of life can be difficult to predict, as the trajectory is often non-linear and can be complicated by inter-current illness or the extent of other chronic conditions. The Gold Standards Framework (Thomas 2003) is a useful aid for identifying people who are likely to require palliative care. It includes two general triggers for palliative care and some condition-specific indicators for CKD. The *surprise question* – 'Would I be surprised if this patient were to die within the next 6–12 months?' – is an intuitive one which draws on the experience of the practitioner and their knowledge of the patient and their circumstances. If the answer to the question is no, it provides an impetus to initiate a number of activities depending on the likely prognosis and the anticipated time frame. The second trigger occurs when a patient expresses a wish to stop 'curative' treatment. The third trigger refers to kidney-specific indicators of advanced disease and includes patients with stage 4 or 5 CKD whose condition is deteriorating with at least two of the following indicators:

- blood results indicating that the patient would normally require dialysis, or blood results on dialysis that are consistently suboptimal
- weight loss of more than 10% in 6 months
- hypoalbuminaemia (<24 g/L)
- complex symptoms that are difficult to control
- requires assistance with mobilising, e.g. walking frame, and in bed for ≥50% of the time
- two or more non-elective admissions in previous three months
- patient has expressed a desire to stop treatment

In addition, certain stages in the patient's care pathway can trigger professionals to review a patient's palliative care needs:

- at time of decision for conservative kidney management
- around decision to withdraw from dialysis
- deteriorating despite dialysis
- time of crisis, e.g. stroke, malignancy
- other life threatening condition, e.g. malignancy
- changing renal replacement modalities due to access failure or ineffective clearance, including a failing transplant

Managing care

For the purposes of organising health care, patients approaching the end of their lives with kidney disease can be broadly divided into three categories – those who:

(1) choose a non-dialytic pathway
(2) decide to withdraw from dialysis
(3) are on dialysis but are generally deteriorating

Decision support

Even in patients with advanced kidney disease, it is important to remember that acute decline may not be due to their kidney injury and may potentially be reversible, depending on the cause. Possible interventions must be considered in light of the patient's general condition prior to any acute illness, as well as their capacity to benefit. This is not always obvious in chronic illness and sometimes requires a 'leap of faith' with circumscribed parameters (specialists are more experienced in this approach). About a quarter of patients receiving RRT will choose to withdraw from dialysis, and most will die within 2–4 weeks of dialysis being stopped. These patients should be given the opportunity to talk through their situation and their reasons for wishing to stop dialysis. This is best done with their specialist team, who are likely to know them well. Ideally, discussions should occur over a period of time during which options can be discussed and re-discussed, giving the patient the time to share their thoughts and any decisions with their immediate family. Professionals may need to facilitate these discussions with the family, and will also need time to establish the patient's needs and wishes, which the patient may not always be able to articulate. Patients with cognitive impairment are sometimes not in a position to decide for themselves whether to withdraw from dialysis; however, multidisciplinary specialist teams are often ideally placed to recognise the clinical or global deterioration and a reduction in quality of life of these people. They will often initiate discussions with the patient's family and advise about prognosis. The point at which the benefits of dialysis are likely outweighed by the physical, psychological and social burden of the treatment is particular to each individual, and should be discussed appropriately with the patient and his or her family.

The focus of care at this stage will move towards symptom control and keeping the patient comfortable. Psychological, social and spiritual needs should be reviewed at regular intervals, and specialist services often include this as part of their multidisciplinary working. In situations where it is obvious that the patient's condition is terminal or the clinician considers it to be, it is important to ensure that the prognosis is shared with the patient and the family. Often this requires the clinician to be explicit in ensuring that the patient and the family understand the gravity of the situation. In patients with CKD the illness trajectory is often characterised by episodes of acute illness and/or deterioration and periods where the patient may be relatively well and stable. It is often difficult during the times of acute illness to know whether the patient will recover from it, particularly if they have recovered from similar episodes before. In situations of uncertainty, it is often necessary to reiterate the possibility that the patient may not recover, and that if they do, they may not be as well as they were before the acute episode. These conversations can help the patient and their family to plan for different eventualities, and can encourage them to articulate their anxieties and needs for which support can be provided.

Terminology

End-of-life care

This is a broad term that identifies more than the phase immediately prior to death. It may be difficult to identify when a patient is at the beginning of this phase, and patient, carer and professional perspectives are likely to differ. This phase is variable and may last for weeks or months. The presence of other acute or chronic conditions can impact on the rate at which kidney function declines. Recognising that a person is entering this phase enables the supportive and palliative care needs of both the patient and the family to be assessed and organised through to the last phase of life and into bereavement. Care should be taken to ensure that the patient and family are aware of, and understand, the likely prognosis. In situations where uncertainties exist around the illness trajectory and time lines, this should be conveyed to the patient and family as appropriate. A common complaint amongst bereaved relatives is that they were unaware of the possibility that the patient could die. Whilst it is sometimes difficult to be accurate over timings, in patients who continue to deteriorate despite appropriate interventions it is important to check with the patient and the family their understanding of the situation and possible outcomes. Most dying patients appreciate the opportunity to make arrangements and put their affairs in order.

Supportive care

Supportive care can be described as care that 'helps the patient and their family to cope with their condition and treatment of it – from pre-diagnosis, through the process of diagnosis and treatment, to cure, continuing illness or death and into bereavement. It helps the patient to maximise the benefits of treatment and to live as well as possible with the effects of the disease. It is given equal priority alongside diagnosis and treatment' (National Council for Palliative Care 2012).

Palliative care

Palliative care is the active holistic care of patients with an advanced and progressive illness. The key aim of palliative care is to deliver the best quality of care to patients by managing any symptoms and providing psychological, social and spiritual support. Palliative care also incorporates the principles of supportive care, and the terms are often used synonymously.

Conservative management

Conservative management (CM) refers to the treatment of advanced kidney disease without dialysis. This includes interventions to slow down or arrest any deterioration of kidney function and to minimise associated complications. Approximately 15–20% of patients with stage 5 CKD will opt for non-dialytic treatment and will be managed on a CM pathway (Murtagh & Sheerin 2010). CM may be the most suitable option for frail patients who already experience a high disease burden and functional decline. For this cohort of patients, the rigours of dialysis and the associated restrictions on daily life can often outweigh any perceived benefits of dialysis. As yet, there is no convincing evidence to suggest that, in older, frail patients, who may have other chronic conditions and general functional impairment, dialysis confers any additional benefit above CM in terms of longevity and quality of care. CM can also be an appropriate option for patients with a kidney transplant whose function is deteriorating and who are clinically unsuitable for, or unwilling to undertake, dialysis or a further transplant. There will also be a group of patients with functioning transplants who are dying from other conditions in which their kidney condition is not considered an issue.

A large proportion of people with CKD experience other, linked, conditions, and this proportion increases with age. The complications of CKD include:

- cardiovascular disease
- mineral and bone disorders (e.g. calcium and phosphate disorders)
- anaemia
- malnutrition
- depression
- increased risk of other non-cardiovascular disease, e.g. infection and cancer
- increased risk of fracture

The relationship between cardiovascular disease and CKD is strong and increases with age. Kidney function in many elderly patients with CKD remains stable, and most will die from cardiovascular events rather than progressing to advanced kidney disease. The impact of additional chronic conditions and general wellbeing may play an important role in patients deciding on their future treatment and whether they are likely to be offered dialysis.

Patient population

People dying with or from kidney disease can be broadly divided into three main groups. The purpose of defining these groups is to anticipate the general trajectory of decline and to ensure services are in place to meet their needs.

The three groups will generally be under the care of specialist services, although there are always exceptions, and irrespective of where the patient is treated, renal services encourage enquiries from those managing patients with CKD in other services:

(1) **Patients clinically unsuitable for or unwilling to undertake dialysis**. This group is usually managed in a CM programme by a specialist team. There is an increasing number of older patients with poor but stable kidney function, who may be discharged back for management in primary care. Clinicians may refer back for specialist management or contact the specialist team for advice should the patient's function deteriorate further. Best practice guidelines are provided by the Renal Association.

(2) **Patients who withdraw from dialysis**. Approximately 25% of patients on maintenance dialysis die following withdrawal from dialysis. In some instances, after years on dialysis and the accumulation of a number of dialysis-related disorders, a patient will choose to stop dialysis.

(3) **Patients who are deteriorating despite dialysis**. Even in those people who are young and fit when they start dialysis, over the years the treatment imposes a high physical and psychological toll and is life-limiting. Similarly, many patients commencing dialysis are older, and they often have a number of other chronic conditions which are likely to deteriorate over time. Despite dialysis, many of these patients decline, and it is important to review these patients independently of their kidney function.

Deciding whether to dialyse or not – a supported decision

Patients with CKD require timely information regarding their prognosis and treatment options in order to make a decision on their preferred treatment pathway. Discussions around treatment modalities should be initiated around a year before the patient requires dialysis. Patients reviewed in the CKD service have usually been attending the clinic for many years. This allows a therapeutic relationship to develop between the patient and the CKD multidisciplinary team and assists the team in anticipating when RRT will be required and when it is appropriate to commence discussions around treatment options.

Determining when a patient will require RRT relies heavily on the clinical knowledge and skills of the specialist team in predicting the rate at which the patient's renal function is declining. The rate of decline is influenced by many factors, including the primary cause of kidney impairment and any infections or related illnesses. The patient's estimated glomerular filtration rate (eGFR) is an arbitrary marker of when to start dialysis, and whilst historically a level of 15 or less was generally used as an indicator, the growing body of evidence from CM clinics suggests that many patients, particularly older ones, can tolerate much lower levels and remain relatively symptom-free.

Decision making around CM is both challenging and difficult and is likely to become more so, as increasing numbers of people survive into old age with the associated increase in the prevalence of chronic conditions. Palliative and supportive components of care are becoming increasingly important in the overall care of the older patient with CKD, who often has limited life expectancy and a high symptom burden. Discussions and any decisions should be carefully documented in the patient record and shared with appropriate stakeholders such as the general practitioner (GP). With the patient's consent, the patient's next of kin should be involved in these discussions. They are often an invaluable support to the patient, and it is important that they understand how the decision was reached, i.e. in the best interests of the patient rather than as a resource issue. In frail patients with complex health needs, their kidney function may be less of an issue than, for example, their heart failure. In these situations, dialysis can often hasten death rather than prolong life. In patients who are clinically unsuitable for dialysis and unlikely to benefit it should not be presented as an option. The reasons for this should be explained at an early stage in the process.

Patients who have decided on a CM pathway can sometimes worry that they have made the wrong decision. It is therefore important to provide ongoing support and reassurance to the patient and the family. Although RRT has transformed the prognosis of renal disease, quality of life remains impaired by the disease and there is a significant treatment burden associated with dialysis. Dialysis is a demanding treatment, even for younger and fitter patients. Some will feel that without any corresponding benefit the burden is too much to tolerate.

Patients may choose not to have dialysis for a number of reasons:

(1) **Feeling too old**. Patients report that if they had been younger they might have opted for dialysis, but many think they have reached a point in their lives where they do not feel they could cope with the arduous nature of dialysis and the impact on their quality of life.
(2) **Difficulty in travelling to the dialysis unit three times a week**. The strain of having to travel to a dialysis unit three times per week is often too much for older and frailer patients. It includes very early starts and lots of waiting around for hospital transport. Other patients return home late at night.
(3) **Feeling well on medication**. Some patients feel their symptoms are well controlled on medication alone and do not think dialysis will offer any additional benefit.
(4) **Not wanting to burden their family**. Having dialysis may result in patients becoming more dependent on their families, for example with household chores and transportation to and from the dialysis unit. Many patients do not want to become a burden on their families.

Conservative management

Conservative management (CM) is a non-dialytic 'active' treatment pathway for people with advanced CKD. The aim of CM is to optimise the quality of life through the control of symptoms and, where possible, the preservation of kidney function (adequately controlling blood pressure can prevent further glomerular damage and slow down the rate of decline in renal function). Patients with stage 5 CKD managed conservatively have significant symptom control needs. Symptoms include lack of energy/fatigue and pruritus, drowsiness, dyspnoea, swelling of the legs, pain, dry mouth, muscle cramps, difficulty concentrating, difficulty sleeping, constipation, skin changes and dizziness. Assessment of symptoms using a generic symptom assessment instrument helps to ensure appropriate management, and adherence to treatment is essential in order to reduce symptom burden. Refer to the Renal Association clinical guidelines for optimising symptom management in conservative management (Farrington & Warwick 2009).

Most patients with low eGFRs are managed through a CM clinic in secondary care, although those with stable kidney function may be discharged back to primary care for monitoring. The number of patients opting for CM is likely to increase in the future as the population ages and there is a rise in the incidence and prevalence of chronic conditions. CM pathways focus on the timely evaluation of prognoses, information streams and discussions around needs and available options, as well as the early identification and management of any symptoms associated with advanced kidney disease. Emotional support, information sharing, goal setting and problem solving are required to engage patients in planning and managing their own care, including, as appropriate, their end-of-life care. Facilitating the delivery of care across multiple providers requires effective communication and is central to the success of this approach.

Ongoing medical care for patients opting not to dialyse

Patients and their families often benefit from the ongoing contact and support of their renal team, and most renal services have arrangements to facilitate this. CM patients are usually reviewed every 2-3 months, as the primary aim is to allow the patient as much time away from hospital as possible. Good practice involves sending a letter to the patient's GP notifying them that the patient has been added to the CM register. It will include a request to include the patient on the practice's palliative care register. In some instances the request will be accompanied by guidelines for end-of-life care in patients with CKD, including advice on pain and symptom management. The guidelines have subsequently been developed into 'Ten Top Tips' for GPs (see NHS Kidney Care website), but they are also relevant to other staff caring for patients with CKD in secondary care.

Patients with kidney disease frequently have other chronic conditions such as diabetes and heart disease and can attend numerous appointments, resulting in excessive time being spent in a hospital environment. Often these specialties work in isolation. This fragmented approach to healthcare delivery can leave patients approaching the end of life feeling vulnerable, with carers having to coordinate services and navigate a range of health and social care systems. Identifying a key worker, such as a case manager, can promote collaborative working between different professionals and services. Using the patient's management plan as a coordinating tool can promote patient-centred care by improving communication and continuity of care. When hospital appointments become more difficult for patients, shared care is an option, whereby the management responsibility is divided between the specialist team and primary care, usually the GP and community nurses. This package of care has been implemented in some areas, with success measured by positive feedback from patients and improved communication between providers. The patient's management plan should to be agreed by all care providers to ensure individual roles and responsibilities are acknowledged. The community nurses usually assess the patient at home and obtain the requested blood tests. The results of these tests are usually reviewed by the CKD nurse specialist, and appropriate changes are made to the patient's care plan or medication regimen. Any changes are relayed to the patient, GP and community nursing team so that they can update their records.

Withdrawing from dialysis

Patients who have been on dialysis for some time often acquire a number of dialysis-related conditions such as heart failure or hypertension due to prolonged fluid overload. In addition, the burden of treatment as well as everyday lifestyle restrictions (such as limitations on diet and fluid intake) can become unbearable after a number of years, and some patients ask for their dialysis to be stopped. This can be a difficult discussion for both patients and staff, with many patients 'not wanting to let their doctor down by stopping dialysis'. Once dialysis is discontinued there is a faster trajectory to death than for patients in the CM group, with death typically occurring over days or weeks. It is usual for a series of meetings to take place between the specialist team, the patient and the family. In situations where the patient is managed at home, district nurses, the patient's GP and the Macmillan team are often involved. This allows for the palliative and supportive needs of the patient to be planned, and offers time for the patient and family to make any necessary arrangements with regard to end-of-life preferences and any legal processes. Dialysis may be continued until appropriate support services are in place.

Patients on long term dialysis whose general health is in persistent decline

The dialysis population is ageing, and with this comes an increased prevalence of chronic conditions, both of which contribute to a patient's overall wellbeing and life expectancy. Dialysis is not a panacea, even for those patients with single-organ disease, and patients will eventually continue to deteriorate due to the progression of other chronic conditions, with or without additional problems associated with long-term dialysis and ageing (for instance mobility and memory problems). Dialysis in itself is life-limiting, and over years patients often become increasingly dependent as they become older and increasingly frail. The insidious onset and persistence of this deterioration may not always be evident in busy outpatient dialysis settings. Regular global assessments and discussions with the patient, the family and any other services involved in care of the patient are often useful in qualifying why dialysis should be continued or when treatment decisions should be revisited. So too is the application of the Gold Standards Framework. If a patient does make a decision to withdraw from dialysis, withdrawal can be planned for a time that best suits the patient and significant others. For example, dialysis might continue until home care services are arranged to allow the patient to be discharged home to die. Any such planning requires ongoing discussions between the patient, the family and the clinical team.

Aims of care management

The aims of care management for people dying with or from CKD are no different from the rest of the population, which is generally to live whatever time is left, optimally. This involves being able to make choices about how to spend that time and where. As well as managing the clinical aspects of palliative care, health services should be aimed at facilitating and supporting choice and providing psychosocial support.

Advance care planning

Advance care planning is a process of discussions between an individual and their care provider, and it takes place in the context of chronic or serious illness in which it is acknowledged that at some point the patient's condition will deteriorate and their capacity to make decisions, and/or their ability to communicate their wishes to others, may recede. An advance care plan (ACP) discussion might include:

- an individual's concerns
- important values or personal goals for care
- understanding about their illness and prognosis
- preferences for types of care or treatment that may be beneficial in the future, and the availability of these

An ACP should be drawn up with a team member competent in the assessment processes with knowledge of available local service providers and support services. The multidisciplinary team, including social workers, counsellors and the palliative care team, should have access to the ACP as necessary. The ACP should be kept by the patient. It should:

- give details of a nominated key worker
- summarise the person's preferences and the choices they wish to make, including their views on resuscitation

- give details of the assessment and the rationale behind decisions, and record the individual needs of carers
- be reviewed regularly
- provide a record of ongoing assessments, outcome of multidisciplinary team meetings and communication with primary care and palliative care services
- be available to all who have a legitimate reason for access, including out-of-hours services and emergency services

End-of-life care tools

There is an increasing number of resources to assist in the assessment, documentation and review of patients with supportive and palliative care needs during the end-of-life care phase. They include the use of palliative care registers which are part of the Quality and Outcomes Framework (QOF), the Gold Standards Framework (GSF), the Preferred Priorities for Care (PPC) advance care plan, and the use of an integrated care pathway such as the Liverpool Care Pathway for the Dying Patient (LCP). These national initiatives are effectively complemented by a growing body of work developed locally, such as the North Bristol guidelines for end-of-life care (North Bristol NHS Trust 2008).

'Cause for concern' register

Increasingly in specialist units a 'cause for concern' register is used to identify those patients who are potentially approaching the end-of-life phase. It promotes a consistent and proactive approach in identifying and supporting patients and staff to facilitate effective communication and care planning in all areas of end-of-life care. The register also facilitates regular review by the multidisciplinary team and links to the palliative care registers held by GPs, and other coordinating aids.

Many patients welcome the opportunity to discuss candidly their condition and prognosis, but others will not. Clinicians are typically sensitive to cues and will not press patients into discussing issues when they are not ready. It is important to consider this aspect of care as an ongoing process, not an event. Establishing a shared view of the person's current situation and likely prognosis between the patient, the family and carers, and among members of the multidisciplinary team, is necessary before moving on to develop care plans relating to future wishes and preferences for end-of-life care. Achieving this can take time, and it should be regularly revisited to ensure that the information remains current.

The Gold Standards Framework

The Gold Standards Framework (GSF) is a useful tool in providing a systematic and standardised approach to delivering high-quality end-of-life care in primary and community settings. Proactive care planning and timely management of symptoms can enhance quality of life for patients, families and carers and help to prevent crises and unscheduled hospital admissions. The GSF highlights the importance of primary care teams working collaboratively with palliative care providers and emphasises the importance of effective communication, coordination and continuity of care. It reinforces the importance of:

- case identification
- holistic assessment
- care planning
- individual case discussions and case management by a multidisciplinary team
- family and carers assessment and support

Preferred Priorities for Care (PPC)

Preferred Priorities for Care is an example of an ACP in which patients can document their preferences and priorities for care during the end-of-life care phase. The PPC document is a patient-held record and can be used as a mechanism to coordinate activities between different providers. The PPC approach aims to help patients to prepare for the future by encouraging and assisting them to think and talk about an area of care that is often not discussed. Not all individuals will be involved in these discussions, but all should have the opportunity to do so. Patients who have a PPC or an ACP document should have this identified in their primary, secondary and out-of-hours records in order for all teams to be aware of the patient's wishes and needs.

Liverpool Care Pathway (LCP)

The LCP is an integrated care pathway designed for the care of patients who are in the last days/hours of their life. The LCP has specific guidelines in the form of treatment algorithms for various symptoms associated with end of life. A modified version is available for use in patients with advanced kidney disease. In particular, it provides a useful guide to managing pain in people with CKD. The risk of toxicity and side effects associated with opioids increases as the level of kidney function decreases. It is necessary to ensure appropriate pain relief for the patient while limiting serious and potentially preventable adverse effects such as respiratory depression, hypotension or central nervous system toxicity, from either the parent drug or its metabolites. The LCP aims to facilitate effective planning and provision of care at the end of life, including symptom control, communication and spiritual or religious needs. Regular review of the LCP by the multidisciplinary team is recorded using a single document. It is recommended that the LCP or its equivalent is implemented in all care settings for patients dying with or from advanced kidney disease. The pathway continues after death, aiming to ensure good communication and care for the family and carers.

Trajectories of decline

Patterns of general decline have been identified in patients with renal disease:

- A **uraemic death** is where patients are managed without dialysis and remain fairly stable over a period of time which can last for months to years. On entering the end-of-life care phase these patients decline relatively quickly over a period of weeks to death. Many of these patients remain in reasonably good health until experiencing a steep decline in the last few weeks of their life. Those patients who withdraw from dialysis usually die from uraemia around 14 days after stopping dialysis.
- A **non-uraemic death** is where patients die from another illness such as cancer or heart disease. Here the trajectory to death is usually predictable, and once the approach to end of life is identified, death can often be planned for and managed.
- **Unknown cause of death** is where it is unclear why death has occurred. Some patients die relatively unexpectedly, or have received inappropriate treatment very close to death, making it difficult to assess the cause of death.

Healthcare professionals in a range of clinical settings are required to identify and treat appropriately any acute or chronic deterioration in patients with CKD. Sometimes this will involve the identification and treatment of inter-current illnesses. Early recognition and initiation of treatment is likely to improve symptom control and may arrest or slow down any deterioration in renal function. Vigilant monitoring of patients is required, as they are vulnerable to opportunistic infections such as pneumonia. Inter-current illness can indicate and accelerate terminal decline in patients with CKD. Treatment of acute illness should be considered in the context of the patient's general condition and their likely response.

Care in the last few days/hours of life and after death

High-quality care at the end of life is achieved through shared decision making and clear communication which acknowledges the values and preferences of individual patients and their families. The characteristics of care during the last days of life that have consistently been found to be important from the patient's perspective are receiving adequate pain and symptom management, avoiding inappropriate prolongation of dying, achieving a sense of control, relieving the burden on loved ones, and strengthening relationships with loved ones. Recording of resuscitation status is useful, but if this has not been discussed previously there is no need to initiate discussion at this stage. During the last days and hours of life patients consistently report that they do not wish to be subjected to interventions with minimal, if any, potential for prolonging life. In this context communications indicating the intention to allow a 'natural death' may be more appropriate than 'do not resuscitate' orders.

Rapid access to care

Rapid access to end-of-life care is important to prevent inappropriate emergency admissions to hospital or initiation of inappropriate therapies such as dialysis. This is most important in those patients who do not have an ACP or PPC in place. In these instances the importance of careful, timely assessment cannot be overemphasised.

In such circumstances, if the patient and/or family express a wish to be cared for at home, then use may be made of the rapid discharge pathway for care of the dying. The pathway allows patients to die in their preferred place of care. It empowers staff to manage complex discharges in the last hours and days of life and encourages cross-sector working. Prior to the development of this pathway it is most likely that these patients would have died in hospital. There is a significant difference between patients' preferences for where they should die and their actual place of death. Most would probably prefer to die at home, but only around 18% do so, with a further 17% dying in care homes and 4% in hospices. Around 58% of all deaths still occur in the acute hospital setting.

There will be a need for timely access to medication and equipment, including out-of hours provision. The role of the key worker is important in ensuring that effective operational links have been established with all services involved in end-of-life care including primary care, community, out-of-hours, palliative care and the ambulance services.

Delivery of high-quality care across all locations

End-of-life care of people with advanced kidney disease needs to be delivered in a range of locations at different stages of the care pathway and in response to changing circumstances. A range of agencies need to work together if patient and carer experience is to be optimised. The needs of individuals are often intensified during this phase of advanced kidney disease, and often added to by the presence of other comorbid conditions. Health and social care professionals addressing these needs must work as a team so that support is coordinated and consistent. This can often entail sharing responsibilities and transferring skills, but maintaining clarity of leadership for the patient and family is essential. In addition to the role of the key worker, senior clinical leadership (medical and nursing) is needed to ensure joint working across organisational, cultural and professional boundaries to deliver high-quality, seamless care whatever the setting. In most instances this will be the patient's home or another community setting. Services should be delivered as locally as possible. At an organisational level, hospital-based kidney care team members with responsibilities for end-of-life care need to work with patient and carer representatives.

Involving and supporting carers

It is important to recognise that the family, including close friends and informal carers, have an important role in the care of people with CKD and may have been supporting and caring for the patient for many years. However, it is likely to be the only time they have been involved in caring for someone who is dying. These key people may well have developed a close relationship with members of the renal team and rely on the team to provide information about the likely progress of the person's condition. The enormous contribution of families and carers often goes unrecognised, but it should be formally acknowledged and they should be offered sensitive and timely information and support that includes:

- Information about the likely progression of the patient's condition. Time scales may be difficult to predict, but it is important for the carer to able to gauge how long they will be able to sustain a certain level of commitment, which is often in the context of work and family commitments.
- Information about services which are available locally to them.
- Practical and emotional support both during the patient's life and following their death.

Practical issues

- Does the patient, the family and the healthcare providers know that the patient is approaching end of life?
- Have discussions or decisions regarding preferences for care been documented, or do they need to be initiated?
- Has the patient and/or family been asked about any spiritual, religious or cultural needs?
- Have all unnecessary investigations and monitoring been discontinued (e.g. blood pressure monitoring and blood tests)?
- Has all non-palliative medication been discontinued?
- Has care provision been organised for comfort (e.g. skin and mouth care)?
- Has the palliation medication been prescribed in a suitable format for administration, and is it accessible should the patient need it?

(Adapted from North Bristol NHS Trust 2008).

Clinical management

The evidence for optimising the clinical management of patients dying with CKD is well documented, and a list of useful resources is included alongside the references at the end of this chapter. We have included here a brief overview of commonly experienced symptoms and treatments in patients with CKD. Medications should be pre-emptively prescribed, and should include a subcutaneous option, on an 'as required' basis, even if the patient is currently asymptomatic. Many of the drugs can be mixed and administered via a syringe driver if necessary. In some areas end-of-life medications are 'pre-packaged', prescribed and stored in the patient's home for use when necessary by the district nurses.

Symptom management

Patients with kidney disease experience many symptoms which can have a negative effect on their wellbeing. Patients may also carry a heavy symptom burden from other medical conditions such as heart failure or diabetes. Good symptom management requires a focus on the symptoms rather than on the presence of individual chronic conditions. The extent of interventions to manage these symptoms will depend upon how troublesome they are to the patient and how close the patient is to death. Common symptoms include:

- **Pain** – Patients should be prescribed a strong opioid to be administered as required. A 'stepwise' approach is recommended, the schedule of which will be dependent upon whether the patient is opioid-naive and whether the pain is intermittent or not. Fentanyl is usually the drug of choice, as it is less toxic for patients with kidney disease. In addition, adjuvant drugs may be used for specific indications – such as midazolam for anxiety and non-steroidal anti-inflammatory drugs (NSAIDs) for joint pain. As symptoms escalate and death approaches, some symptoms, such as fluid overload, become difficult to treat, indicating the approach of the end of life. Any problems associated with optimising symptom management should be referred to the specialist or palliative care team involved.
- **Restlessness and agitation** – Midazolam can be used PRN or included in a syringe driver. Restless legs is a common symptom in patients with kidney disease, and clonazepam, levodopa, amitriptyline or gabapentin can be effective in treating this.
- **Excessive secretions** – Hyoscine butylbromide can be given subcutaneously, intermittently or as an infusion.
- **Pruritis** – Although managing pruritis effectively is difficult, it is worth persisting with as it can make life miserable for patients. Treatment may include the use of an emollient if the skin is dry. If it is widespread, terfenadine may be used. Itchiness that disrupts sleep can be treated with a sedating antihistamine such as chlorphenamine. Ondansetron has also been used but should be used with caution (Murtagh & Weisbord 2010).
- **Breathlessness** – Sit the patient upright and apply a cool fan. Administer oxygen if saturations are low and if the patient can tolerate it. Comfort and reassure the patient and the family. Administer a strong opioid as necessary (usually a lesser dose than is used for management of pain). If the patient is

breathless because they are anxious or frightened, a benzodiazepine such as midazolam can be used. In some instances, the patient's breathlessness may be due to fluid overload, which can be very distressing. The above interventions may be instigated, as well as sublingual nitrates. In patients who still pass urine, high-dose furosemide may be useful, or in some instances a unit of blood may be removed through venesection.

- **Nausea and vomiting** – If oral administration is ineffective or not possible, antiemetics can be administered subcutaneously intermittently or over 24 hours via a syringe driver.

Conclusion

High-quality end-of-life care is important for everyone. In supporting patients dying with CKD and their families, patients who are deteriorating need to be identified as such. Regular ongoing needs assessments and discussions with patients and families allows care to be proactively organised. An individualised management plan, held by the patient and a nominated key worker, helps to facilitate effective communication and coordination of care across different providers. A number of evidence-based guidelines and pathways, alongside increased access to shared care programmes, mean that patients are no longer restricted to specialist services and secondary care to ensure they receive the care they need.

References and resources

Department of Health (2005) *National Service Framework for Renal Services. Part Two: Chronic Kidney Disease, Acute Renal Failure and End of Life Care*. http://www.dh.gov.uk/en/Publicationsandstatistics/Publications/PublicationsPolicyAndGuidance/DH_4101902 (accessed September 2012).

Edinburgh Royal Infirmary Renal Unit (Edren). http://www.edren.org (accessed September 2012).

Farrington, K., & Warwick, G. (2009) End of life care: conservative kidney management and withdrawal of dialysis. In: Planning, initiating and withdrawal of renal replacement therapy, Guidelines 6.1–6.5. Renal Association. http://www.renal.org/clinical/guidelinessection/RenalReplacementTherapy.aspx (accessed September 2012).

Gold Standards Framework. http://www.goldstandardsframework.org.uk (accessed September 2012).

Liverpool Care Pathway for the Dying Patient (LCP). http://www.mcpcil.org.uk (accessed September 2012).

Murtagh, F. & Sheerin, N.(2010) Conservative management of end-stage renal disease. In: *Supportive Care for the Renal Patient*, 2nd edition (ed. E.J. Chambers, E.A. Brown & M.J. Germain), pp. 253–68. Oxford University Press, Oxford.

Murtagh, F. & Weisbord, S.D. (2010) Symptoms in renal disease: their epidemiology, assessment, and management. In: *Supportive Care for the Renal Patient*, 2nd edition (ed. E.J. Chambers, E.A. Brown & M.J. Germain), pp. 103–38. Oxford University Press, Oxford.

NHS End of Life Care Programme. Preferred Priorities for Care (PPC). http://www.endoflifecareforadults.nhs.uk/tools/core-tools/preferredprioritiesforcare (accessed September 2012).

NHS Kidney Care. Palliative and end of life care in advanced kidney disease. http://www.kidneycare.nhs.uk/our_work_programmes/_palliative_and_end_of_life_care_in_advanced_kidney_disease (accessed September 2012).

NICE (2011) *Chronic kidney disease*. Clinical Guideline 73. National Institute for Health and Clinical Excellence, London. http://www.nice.org.uk/CG73 (accessed September 2012).

North Bristol NHS Trust (2008) Supportive care: end of life phase. Guidelines for health care professionals in the care of patients with established renal failure who are in the last days of life. http://www.nbt.nhs.uk/clinicians/services-referral/renal-kidney-gps/supportive-care-guidelines (accessed September 2012).

National Council for Palliative Care (2012) Palliative care explained. http://www.ncpc.org.uk/palliative-care-explained (accessed September 2012).

Renal Association. http://www.renal.org (accessed September 2012).

Stein, A. & Wild, J. (2002) *Kidney Failure Explained*, 2nd edition. Class Publishing. London.

Thomas, K. (2003) The Gold Standards Framework in community palliative care. *European Journal of Palliative Care*, **10**, 113-15.

Index

Kidney Disease Management: A Practical Approach for the Non-Specialist Healthcare Practitioner, First Edition. Edited by Rachel Lewis and Helen Noble.
© 2013 John Wiley & Sons, Ltd. Published 2013 by John Wiley & Sons, Ltd.